T0309573

Management of Knee Osteoarthritis in the Younger, Active Patient

David A. Parker

Editor

Management of Knee Osteoarthritis in the Younger, Active Patient

An Evidence-Based Practical Guide for Clinicians

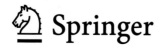

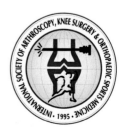

Editor
David A. Parker
Sydney Orthopaedic Research Institute
Sydney
New South Wales
Australia

ISBN 978-3-662-48528-6   ISBN 978-3-662-48530-9   (eBook)
DOI 10.1007/978-3-662-48530-9

Library of Congress Control Number: 2015959845

Springer Heidelberg New York Dordrecht London
© ISAKOS 2016

Printed on acid-free paper

Springer-Verlag GmbH Berlin Heidelberg is part of Springer Science+Business Media (www.springer.com)

Preface

As clinicians, how do we manage the 45-year-old man who has symptomatic articular cartilage wear but wants to continue with his sports or the 35-year-old woman who is having trouble with her normal daily activities due to post-meniscectomy arthritis? Increasingly commonly, physicians are facing these management problems: younger, active patients who are developing osteoarthritis which is impinging on the activities that they want or need to do. Management of these patients is a major challenge and will always involve a balance between optimising function and keeping expectations realistic. To be able to provide such patients with optimal advice and management, the physician or allied health professional needs to have a comprehensive knowledge of the condition, its natural history, the various treatment options available, and the evidence base for each. This text has been created in order to provide clinicians with the knowledge and resources to provide patients with such a wholistic, optimal management plan to maximise each patient's function and quality of life.

This new text comprehensively covers all areas relevant to the management of osteoarthritis and localised articular cartilage pathology in younger patients who are still wishing to maintain a high level of physical activity and exercise. The earlier chapters address the basic science behind osteoarthritis, including the definition, classification, and epidemiology and natural history of the condition. A clear understanding of this is obviously critical to its management. The aetiology of osteoarthritis is also discussed, particularly distinguishing between modifiable and non-modifiable risk factors and their relevance to management. The subsequent chapter discusses the many non-surgical treatment modalities available for osteoarthritis. In particular, each treatment is discussed with special reference to the relevant evidence base, and subsequently the appropriate recommendations for its use are provided. A particular focus is placed on the importance of the multidisciplinary approach to the effective management of osteoarthritis.

The following chapters then address the role of surgical management. This can be divided into techniques that attempt to preserve and possibly restore the native knee joint and those that involve replacement of the joint. All of the available surgical techniques are discussed in detail, once again focusing on the evidence base to support each treatment, and provide the appropriate indications. Equally importantly, the text discusses the clinical scenarios for which surgery is not appropriate. The surgical techniques involved in restoring and retaining the native knee joint that are discussed include meniscal and chondral surgery, arthroscopic debridement, and osteotomy for realignment of the joint. The arthroplasty component of the text covers all areas of prosthetic resurfacing, including localised resurfacing, unicompartmental replacement, and total knee replacement. Of particular significance is the importance of patient selection, technique, and prosthesis selection and providing the appropriate recommendations for levels of activity post-arthroplasty surgery. The longer-term prognosis of arthroplasty in the younger active patient is carefully considered, to provide surgeons with the appropriate information to give their patients accurate advice about their future.

Producing this textbook has involved collaboration between many authors from a number of countries. Authors have been largely selected from the Knee Committee of the International Society for Arthroscopy, Knee Surgery, and Orthopaedic Sports Medicine, with additional contributions from the American Association of Hip and Knee Surgeons for the arthroplasty section of the text. This has brought together an international faculty providing a true global perspective on the topic. The authors have all initially constructed their respective chapters based on a systematic review of the literature, coupled with their own extensive clinical experience and expertise. The authors then all met together over 2 days in the USA in March of 2015 to present their reviews to the entire group for discussion, review, and refinement, which gave each author the opportunity to add contributions as appropriate to each topic. Each author then finalised their chapter for editorial review and subsequent provision to the publisher. The end result is I believe a text that provides a practical and invaluable reference for clinicians managing patients with osteoarthritis, which should ultimately improve the management of these patients, allowing them to remain active and sustain their quality of life. I sincerely hope that you find this text useful in your clinical practice for the management of these patients.

Sydney, Australia   David A. Parker, FRACS

Contents

Part I

Introduction, and Nonoperative Management

Osteoarthritis: Definition, Etiology, and Natural History

1

Elizabeth A. Arendt

Contents

E.A. Arendt, MD
Department of Orthopaedic Surgery,
University of Minnesota, Suite R200, 2450
Riverside Ave. South, Minneapolis, MN 55454, USA
e-mail: arend001@umn.edu

1.1 Definition of Osteoarthritis, Classification, and Epidemiology

Osteoarthritis (OA) is one of the most common causes of disability in adults. The prevalence increases with age, with a surprising 13.9 % of the population over 25 years old being affected and 33.6 % of the population over 65 years old affected [1].

OARSI (Osteoarthritis Research Society International) defines osteoarthritis as "a disorder involving movable joints characterized by cell stress and extracellular matrix degradation initiated by micro- and macro-injury that activates maladaptive repair responses including pro-inflammatory pathways of innate immunity." This in turn manifests initially as abnormal joint tissue metabolism and subsequently by anatomic and physiologic derangements. Clinically, this can present as cartilage degradation, bone remodeling, and osteophyte formation, with joint inflammation, pain, and loss of normal joint function.

The classification of osteoarthritis is varied. Classification strategies include:

1. Classification via radiographic imaging [2]
2. Classification utilizing advanced imaging, including whole-organ scoring [3]
3. Classification emphasizing clinical symptoms, including stiffness, swelling, knee range of motion, and knee crepitus [4]
4. Combination of symptoms and imaging [4]

© ISAKOS 2016
D.A. Parker (ed.), *Management of Knee Osteoarthritis in the Younger, Active Patient:*
An Evidence-Based Practical Guide for Clinicians, DOI 10.1007/978-3-662-48530-9_1

Table 1.1 American College of Rheumatology radiological and clinical criteria for osteoarthritis of the knee [4]

1	Knee pain for most days of previous month
2	Osteophytes at joint margins on radiographs
3	Synovial fluid typical of osteoarthritis (laboratory)
4	Age $\geq$40 years
5	Crepitus on active joint motion
6	Morning stiffness $\leq$30 min duration

Knee osteoarthritis (clinical and radiographic) if 1 and 2; 1, 3, 5, and 6; or 1, 4, 5, and 6 are present

Table 1.2 Advanced imaging for osteoarthritis of the knee

MRI
Standard SPGR
Cartilage morphology quantitative/time-consuming analyses
T2 MRI relaxation
Collagen distribution
Semiquantitative information on cartilage quality/complex interpretation
T1ρ proteoglycan distribution
Semiquantitative information on cartilage quality/complex interpretation
23Na MRI FCD/proteoglycan content
Semiquantitative information on cartilage quality/field strength $\geq$3 T
dGEMRIC FCD/proteoglycan content
Semiquantitative information on cartilage quality, early changes/contrast agent needed

The American College of Rheumatology radiologic and clinical criteria for osteoarthritis of the knee are listed in Table 1.1. For the purposes of this review, osteoarthritis, arthrosis, and arthritis will be used interchangeably.

Although radiographic imaging classification has stood the test of time, the most limiting aspect of this classification is that it often does not detect arthritis until a more advanced stage. Plain radiographs are an imperfect indicator for early arthritis, with a more complete picture of intra-articular disease revealed by other methods, including magnetic resonance imaging (MRI) (Table 1.2) and, more recently, serum and urinary markers looking for bone/cartilage/synovial degradation and/or bone/cartilage/synovial synthesis [5, 6].

In addition to defining and classifying established arthritis, more difficult to define are the following:

1. (a) How does one define "early arthritis"? If you have radiographic and/or imaging signs only, with no correlation to clinical symptoms or objective physical exam signs, is this arthritis?

   (b) Should we define clinical (symptomatic) arthritis separate from radiographic (imaging) arthritis?
2. If there are focal defects, particularly focal defects on only one side of the joint, is this defined as arthritis?
3. Is chondrosis and arthrosis the same disease along a continuum?
4. Should post-traumatic arthrosis and idiopathic arthrosis follow the same disease progression? If these two diseases are separate, then in which category would we place overuse or overload OA?

Classification strategies for radiographic imaging have emphasized joint space narrowing, subchondral sclerosis, and osteophyte formation (Tables 1.3 and 1.4). A recent study assessed the validity and sensitivity to change of three radiographic scales of knee OA [7]. The authors found high validity to assess knee OA severity but only moderate sensitivity to change. The authors recommended caution when using ordinal radiographic grading scales to monitor knee OA over time. Joint axis deviation is a much-used clinical tool, although it is not as frequently used in radiographic classifications. By advanced imaging (MRI), the most common features that indicate osteoarthritis are cartilage thinning and subchondral bone edema. Whole-organ body imaging is largely being used as a research tool only (Table 1.5).

The struggle to define osteoarthritis is compounded when the clinician (or researcher) tries to define arthritis progression. One could define progression based on the classification strategies, i.e., change in radiographic markers (joint space narrowing, osteophyte formation, and/or axis deviation), change in MRI imaging (increase in cartilage thinning, increase in subchondral bone edema,

Table 1.3 Radiographic imaging classification for osteoarthritis of the knee [2]

Kellgren–Lawrence grading system	
Grade 0	No feature of osteoarthritis
Grade 1	Doubtful narrowing of joint space and possible osteophytic lipping
Grade 2	Definite osteophytes and possible narrowing of joint space
Grade 3	Moderate multiple osteophytes, definite narrowing of joint space, and some sclerosis and possible deformity of bone ends
Grade 4	Large osteophytes, marked narrowing of joint space, severe sclerosis, and definite deformity of bone ends

Table 1.4 Clinical assessment of joint axis deviation for osteoarthritis of the knee [18]

Osteoarthritis research society international grading system for medial and lateral tibiofemoral joint space narrowing	
Grade 0	Normal
Grade 1	Mild (1–33 % narrowed)
Grade 2	Moderate (34–66 % narrowed)
Grade 3	Severe (67–100 % narrowed)

Table 1.5 MRI whole-organ scoring for osteoarthritis of the knee

KOSS [19]	Semiquantitative, whole-organ score, time consuming, observer variance
WORMS [20]	Semiquantitative, whole-organ score, time consuming, observer variance
BLOKS [21]	Semiquantitative, whole-organ score, time consuming, observer variance

and/or osteophyte formation), and increase in symptoms of stiffness and swelling best evaluated by a change in patient-reported outcome measure scales. Indeed, thought leaders of the Osteoarthritis Research Society International have called for greater consensus around more sensitive and specific diagnostic criteria for OA to aid in both research and clinical endeavors [8].

This chapter will not answer these questions, but the reader should be apprised that these questions continue to be debated without consensus in our literature. Though clinical knowledge depends on research-directed discoveries, the rigor necessary to answer these questions is different for the clinician and the researcher.

1.2 Etiology

One factor that is consistent in all studies of arthritis is its association with the aging process. The etiology of osteoarthritis has long been thought to be cartilage driven. Imaging definitions of osteoarthritis have as a main factor some inclusion of changes in the subchondral bone. Osteophyte formation, bone remodeling, subchondral sclerosis, and bone attrition are crucial for radiographic diagnosis; several of these bone changes take place not only during the final stages of the disease but sometimes at the onset of the disease, before cartilage degradation is apparent. This adds to the difficulty of using radiographic markers as an indication of the stage of the disease or the stage of potential disease progression. However, findings collectively suggest that the subchondral bone could be the initiator of cartilage damage, and current attention has focused on the role subchondral bone plays in the etiology of osteoarthritis.

Recent evidence shows an additional and integrated role of bone and synovial tissue. Synovial inflammation corresponds to clinical symptoms such as joint swelling and inflammatory pain and is thought to be secondary to cartilage debris and catabolic mediators entering the synovial cavity. Synovial macrophages produce catabolic and pro-inflammatory mediators, leading to inflammation, which starts a negative balance of cartilage matrix degradation and repair. This process, in turn, amplifies synovial inflammation, thus creating a vicious cycle. Inflammation is an important aspect of arthritis, and the degree of inflammation likely varies depending on patient-specific innate factors and local joint factors. This can create a spectrum of clinical presentations for the same imaging picture and varying timelines for disease progression.

1.3 Risk Factors

A review of relevant literature on risk factors is presented in Table 1.6. Pertinent points are discussed below.

Table 1.6 Risk factors for, and etiology of, osteoarthritis of the knee

Study	Topic	Study type	Results
Andriacchi (2015) [22]	Risk factors of knee OA – systems view of pathogenesis	Literature review to develop systems model to predict cartilage thinning at 5-year follow-up	The primary risk factors for OA (aging, obesity, and joint trauma) are associated with systemic biological, mechanical, and structural changes; when one risk factor spikes, the interaction among these systems determines the rate of progression to clinical OA
Evangelou (2015) [23]	Meta-analysis of genome-wide association studies confirms a susceptibility locus for knee osteoarthritis on chromosome 7q22 Etiology: genetics	Meta-analysis of four genome-wide association studies of 2371 cases of knee OA and 35,909 controls in Caucasian populations, with data from ten additional replication data sets	Cumulative sample size of 6709 cases and 44,439 controls. One genome-wide significant locus was identified on chromosome 7q22 for knee OA (rs4730250, $p = 9.2 \text{ Å} \sim 10-9$), thereby confirming its role as a susceptibility locus for OA
Kerkhof (2015) [24]	Prognostic model for knee OA incidence	Risk model + validation, prospective study	The cohorts of three prospective studies were used, each with differing patient characteristics (e.g., only age ≥ 55, only female). Of modest predictive value for OA were genetic score, pain, collagen levels, sex, age, and BMI. The strongest predictive value was minor or doubtful radiographic degenerative features, of a sort that radiologists tend not to report (KL score of 1)
Lo (2015) [25]	Habitual running is not detrimental and may be protective of symptomatic knee OA	Cross-sectional study of 2439 OAI participants using knee XRs, symptoms assessment, and lifetime activity surveys	55 % female, mean age of 64.7, 28 % ran at some time in their life. Exposure to nonelite running at any time in one's lifetime is not associated with higher odds of prevalent knee pain, symptomatic OA, or radiographic OA
Sanghi (2015) [26]	Risk factors of knee OA – diet	Case (180) + control (180)	Low intake of vitamin D and vitamin C is a possible risk factor for OA, especially in females
Yucesoy (2015) [15]	Risk factors of knee OA – occupation and genetics	Literature review (not systematic)	Describes OA in all joints. For knees, a clear occupational risk factor was heavy physical workload. Also of note were vibration, repetitive movement, and long hours of kneeling, squatting, or standing
Apold (2014) [27]	Risk factors for knee replacement – sex as a variable	Prospective 12-year study of 315,495 Norwegians	1323 individuals received knee replacement for primary OA (0.4 %). Independent risk factors were high BMI and heavy labor at work. Rate of knee replacement was double for women (.55) than men (.28). High BMI risk increase in men = 6× and women = 11×. Combining heavy labor with high BMI was particularly hazardous, with risk increase in men = 12× and women = 16×. Smoking had no association in males and a (strangely) positive effect in females
Fanelli (2014) [28]	Follow-up on surgically treated knee dislocations – joint injury as a variable	Case review, minimum 5-year follow-up, 44 cases	At a mean of 10 years post-op (range 5–22 years), dislocated knees treated surgically were stable, but incidence of OA was 23 %. (This study notes that Engebretsen 2009 and Richter 2002 saw OA at 85 %)

Author (Year) [Ref]	Topic	Study design	Findings
Logerstedt (2014) [29]	Moderate and severe knee OA by sex differences – progression and sex	Cross-sectional, 2-year longitudinal, case (226) + control (63)	For moderate OA (only), females had weaker performance scores and higher ADL impairment. No difference in controls or in severe OA
Silverwood (2014) [30]	Risk factors of knee OA – age ≥50	Systematic review + meta-analysis, 46 studies	Risks = overweight/obese, female, previous trauma; n/a smoking, n/a hand OA
Bennell (2013) [10]	Genesis and management of knee OA – role of LE muscle	Extensive literature review from PT perspective	This paper is 32 pages long with 181 references, covering the influence of LE muscle activity on knee joint loading, deficits in muscle function in knee OA, and evidence on the role of muscle in the development and progression of knee OA. Covers muscle activation, proprioception, OA onset and progression, and muscle function deficit intervention and modification. Ample evidence for muscle (particularly quadriceps) strengthening exercises resulting in improvements in pain, physical function, and QOL. Pages 17–22 cover exercise Rx for knee OA
Chundru (2013) [31]	Focal knee lesions in knee pairs for asymptomatic and symptomatic patients	Case + control, radiographic study, 3 T MRI of both knees to assess focal knee lesions	Control = 60 subjects, aged 45–55, with OA risk factors, no radiographic OA, without knee pain; cases = 30. Same demographics with right knee pain; + 30 with bilateral knee pain. Findings: Radiographic focal knee lesions in the right and left knee of subjects with OA risk factors were positively associated with each other. Knee pain is independent of focal lesions
Felson (2013) [9]	OA as a disease of abnormal mechanics Etiology = progression?	Epidemiological literature review, not systematic	Author picks through OA literature to construct three points regarding abnormal mechanics: increased physical forces cause OA; above all other factors, pathomechanics prompt disease progression; and inflammation in OA is a consequence of abnormal mechanics and is almost never primary
Jungmann (2013) [32]	Risk of cartilage degradation – metabolic factors (e.g., high abdominal circumference, hypertension, high fat consumption, and diabetes mellitus)	NIH multicenter, longitudinal, observational cohort	Subjects: no symptomatic radiographic knee OA at baseline but ≥1 risk factor for developing knee OA, with full MRI scans (n=403, aged 45–60). Follow-up MRIs with T2 relaxation data (n=381). Metabolic risk factors of high abdominal circumference, hypertension, high fat consumption, and diabetes mellitus had significant association with higher baseline T2 relaxation times. The cumulative number of metabolic risk factors present in an individual was associated with higher baseline T2 values, independent of BMI
Martin (2013) [33]	Risk factors of knee OA – BMI, occupation, activity level	British 1946 birth cohort; snapshots at age 36, 43, and 53; n=2597	OA association with BMI, strong and manual labor occupation, moderate. High BMI levels more risky for active than sedentary participants. In low BMI women, high activity levels had a protective effect for OA
Prieto-Alhambra (2013) [34]	Incidence and risk factors of OA – age, gender, and crossover sites (knee-hip-hand)	Spain cohort, retrospective, 2006–2010, age ≥40, n=3,266,826	Diagnosis based on ICD-10 code. OA incidence in only the knee = 96,222 (2.95 %), knee + hand = 14,171 (.43 %), knee + hip = 14,585 (.45 %), and all three = 1391 (.04 %). Total knee incidence 3.87 %. Knee-only were highly female (64.4 %), BMI 25–30 (37.86 %)/BMI ≥30 (51.59 %), and comorbid for hypertension (55.47 %). Mean age at diagnosis 67 years; excellent and detailed figures on incidence by age. Crossover of knee ± hip ± hand attenuate when adjusted for BMI

(continued)

Table 1.6 (continued)

Study	Topic	Study type	Results
Boyan (2012) [13]	Sex differences in knee OA	2-page editorial	Letter calling for knee OA studies to factor sex in all research done, because women have increased prevalence of knee OA, greater pain, and more substantial reduction in function and quality of life when disease is present
Hansen (2012) [35]	Running does not cause OA of the hip or knee	Literature review	Low- and moderate-distance running is not associated with OA. Long-distance running is inconclusive. Barefoot and minimalist shoes are inconclusive. Increased risk of developing OA = increasing age, previous joint injury, and greater BMI
Huffman (2012) [14]	OA and the metabolic syndrome: more evidence that the etiology of OA is different in men and women – sex as a variable	Editorial with literature review	3-page article listing 15 studies chosen to illustrate the topic. Independent of the effects of obesity, altered metabolism is related to knee OA, and these relations differ for men and women. Example studies are cited: crossover with hand OA, glucose, hormones, growth factors, transcription factors, nitric oxide-reactive oxygen species, systemic inflammatory markers and mediators, leptin, cholesterol, insulin resistance, and sex differences in fat deposition patterns. Sex differences are noted at epidemiologic, radiographic, circulating biomarker, hormonal, and cellular levels
Palmer (2012) [36]	Risk factors of knee OA – occupational activities	Systematic literature review	43 papers 1948–2011. Table 3 is a huge synopsis of risk sorted by physical activity and study. High-risk occupational activities were squatting/kneeling, lifting, climbing, and heavy work. Particularly deleterious interactions of high BMI with kneeling/squatting and heavy lifting
Sridhar (2012) [37]	Obesity and symptomatic osteoarthritis of the knee	Instructional review	This instructional review paper covers knee OA pathophysiology (mechanical and biochemical), natural history (progression), and treatment (weight loss, TKR)
Yoshimura (2012) [17]	Accumulation of metabolic risk factors (overweight, hypertension, dyslipidemia, impaired glucose tolerance) raises the risk of occurrence and progression of knee OA: a 3-year follow-up of the ROAD study	Epidemiological cohort ($n = 1690$) with 3-year follow-up + radiography ($n = 1384$)	Knee OA defined as KL ≥ 2. Odds ratios for OA metabolic risk factors significantly increased according to the number of MS components present (one = 2.33, two = 2.82, three = 9.83). OA progression risk significantly increased according to the number of MS components present (one = 1.38, two = 2.29, three = 2.80). Metabolic syndrome prevention may be useful in reducing future knee OA risk
Chaganti (2011) [38]	Risk factors for incident osteoarthritis of the hip and knee	Review of literature on multiple factors	There are several modifiable risk factors that have been consistently identified as associated with incident radiographic knee osteoarthritis, in particular obesity, prior knee injury, and repetitive bending

Study	Title	Methods	Findings
Hovis [39] (2011)	Association of exercise and knee-bending activities with MRI-based knee cartilage T2 relaxation times and morphologic abnormalities in asymptomatic subjects from the OAI, with or without OA risk factors	128 subjects with knee OA risk factors and 33 normal control subjects aged 45–55, with a body mass index of 18–27 kg/m² and no knee pain. Subjects were categorized according to exercise level, self-reported frequent knee-bending activities, and WORMS	Subjects without OA risk factors displayed no significant differences in T2 values according to exercise level. Frequent knee-bending activities were associated with higher T2 values in all subjects and with more severe cartilage lesions in the group with OA risk factors. In subjects at risk of knee OA, light exercise was associated with low T2 values, whereas moderate/strenuous exercise in women was associated with high T2 values. Higher T2 values and WORMS grades were observed in frequent knee benders, suggesting greater cartilage degeneration in these individuals
Jones (2011) [40]	Physical activity and knee OA assessed via MRI	Clinical Focus article, literature review	The paper suggests that aerobic and strengthening exercise improves symptoms of OA but has little effect on radiographic structural change in the knee
McWilliams (2011) [12]	Occupational risk factors for osteoarthritis of the knee: a meta-analysis	Studies of knee OA ($n=51$), persistent knee pain ($n=12$), and knee OA progression ($n=3$) were retrieved. Occupational risks for knee OA were examined in a total of 526,343 subjects in 8 cohort/prospective/longitudinal studies, 25 cross-sectional studies, and 18 case–control studies	Study designs showed a positive association between knee OA and occupational activities. Overall, there was evidence of publication bias ($P<0.0001$) which was apparent in the cross-sectional and case–control studies ($P<0.0001$ and $P=0.0247$, respectively). Influences of publication bias and heterogeneity are important limitations of these studies. Prospective studies would greatly improve the evidence base
Molloy (2011) [41]	Contact sports and osteoarthritis	Literature summary (mainly quotes other papers)	Animal and human studies have shown no evidence of increased risk of hip or knee OA with moderate exercise and in the absence of traumatic injury; sporting activity has a protective effect. One age-matched case–control study found that recreational runners who ran 12–14 miles per week for up to 40 years had no increase in radiological or symptomatic hip or knee OA
Muthuri (2011) [42]	History of knee injuries and knee osteoarthritis: a meta-analysis of observational studies	Twenty-four observational studies ($n=20,997$) were included in the meta-analysis of which there were seven cohort, five cross-sectional, and 12 case–control studies	History of knee injury is a major risk factor for the development of knee OA irrespective of study design and definition of knee injury. As one of the few modifiable/preventable risk factors, knee injury should be part of the future prevention program in reducing the risk of knee OA
Muthuri (2011) [43]	Risk reduction in knee osteoarthritis estimated through a meta-analysis of observational studies. Focus on obesity	Meta-analysis of relative risk for knee OA associated with BMI and estimate of potential risk reduction by controlling for BMI. 47 studies ($n=446,219$) were included: 14 cohort, 19 cross-sectional, and 14 case–control studies	Obesity is a risk factor for many conditions, including knee OA. The benefit of modifying this risk factor may cause significant risk reduction of knee OA in the general population, especially in Western countries where obesity is prevalent

(continued)

Table 1.6 (continued)

Study	Topic	Study type	Results
Papavasiliou (2011) [44]	Participation in athletic activities may be associated with later development of hip and knee OA	Literature review	24 papers, of which 15 covered knee OA. Nine studies positive for increased prevalence of knee OA in athletes; no connection in six. Higher-risk sports were endurance and power sports, running, soccer, weight lifting, and football. Most studies had low levels of evidence and methodological weaknesses
Segal (2011) [45]	Quadriceps muscle weakness as a risk for knee OA incidence or progression	Clinical Feature article, literature review	Paper suggests that quadriceps muscle strength training can reduce risk for symptomatic knee OA incidence, although not radiographic incidence. In women, greater quad strength is associated with lower risk for progression of joint space narrowing and cartilage loss
Valdes (2011) [46]	Genetic epidemiology of hip and knee osteoarthritis	Literature review. Genetic studies of patients with OA reviewed for molecular mechanisms responsible for disease manifestations, including joint damage, nociception, and chronic pain	Genome-wide association studies have uncovered a likely role in OA for the genes encoding structural extracellular matrix components (such as DVWA) and molecules involved in prostaglandin metabolism (such as DQB1 and BTNL2). A ~300 kilobase region in chromosome 7q22 is also associated with OA susceptibility
Yusuf (2011) [47]	BMI and alignment and their interaction as risk factors for progression of knees with radiographic signs of OA	Radiographs of 181 knees from 155 patients (85 % female, mean age of 60 years) with radiographic signs of OA were analyzed at baseline and after 6 years	Seventy-six knees (42 %) showed progression: 27 in lateral and 66 in medial compartment. Knees from overweight and obese patients had an increased risk for progression. Overweight is associated with progression of knee OA and shows a small interaction with alignment
Klussman (2010) [48]	Individual and occupational risk factors for knee osteoarthritis: case–control study in Germany	Patients with and without symptomatic knee OA completed a standardized questionnaire. 739 cases and 571 controls	The results support a dose–response relationship between kneeling/squatting and symptomatic knee OA in men and in women. Occupational risks such as jumping or climbing stairs/ladders, as discussed in the literature, did not correlate with symptomatic knee OA in the present study
Sowers (2010) [16]	Review of the literature on the evolving role of obesity in knee OA	Summarizes topic-specific studies	Cytokines associated with adipose tissue, including leptin, adiponectin, and resistin, may influence OA through direct joint degradation or control of local inflammatory processes. Further, pound for pound, not all obesities are equivalent to the development of knee OA; development appears to be strongly related to the coexistence of disordered glucose and lipid metabolism

Stehling (2010) [49]	Prevalence of focal knee abnormalities using 3 T MRI in relation to physical activity levels in asymptomatic, middle-aged subjects from OAI	Analyzed baseline data from 236, 45–55-year-old individuals (136 women, 100 men) without knee pain and a BMI of 19–27 kg/m^2. Physical activity levels were determined in all subjects using PASE. MRI at 3 T was performed	Asymptomatic middle-aged individuals from the OAI incidence cohort had a high prevalence of knee abnormalities; more physically active individuals had significantly more severe knee abnormalities independent of sex, age, BMI, KL score, and OA risk factors
Toivanen (2010) [11]	Obesity, physically demanding work, and traumatic knee injury are the major risk factors for OA	Prospective survey study of 8000 subjects (Finland, age >30) in which 823 patients free of knee OA were identified. 22 years later, re-examined and 94 new OA cases were found	The risk of developing knee OA was strongly associated with BMI (kg/m^2); adjusted for age, sex, and other covariates and compared with the reference category (BMI <25.0). The roles of obesity, heavy workload, and knee injury are strongly associated with the etiology of knee OA
Blagojevic (2009) [50]	Risk factors for OA in elderly adults	Systematic review and meta-analysis; 2223 studies reviewed, 85 included	The main factors consistently associated with knee OA were obesity (pooled OR = 2.63, 95 % CI = 2.28–3.05), previous knee trauma (pooled OR = 3.86, 95 % CI = 2.61–5.70), hand OA (pooled OR = 1.49, 95 % CI = 1.05–2.10), female gender (pooled OR = 1.84, 95 % CI = 1.32–2.55), and older age. Physical occupation and physical activity need more and better quality studies

Abbreviations: *OA* osteoarthritis, *OAI* Osteoarthritis Initiative, *XR* x-ray, *ADL* activities of daily living, *BMI* body mass index, *KL* Kellgren–Lawrence, *NIH* National Institutes of Health, *MRI* magnetic resonance imaging, *ICD* International Classification of Diseases of the World Health Organization, *LE* lower extremity, *PT* physical therapy, *QOL* quality of life, *ROAD* Research on Osteoarthritis/Osteoporosis Against Disability, *MS* metabolic syndrome, *TKR* total knee replacement, *OR* odds ratio, *CI* confidence interval, *OAI* Osteoarthritis Initiative, *PASE* Physical Activity Scale for the Elderly, *WORMS* Whole-Organ MRI Score

1.3.1 Altered Mechanics

Abnormal mechanics can cause OA in both animals and humans. Once OA has developed, abnormal mechanics can overwhelm other factors leading to disease worsening and clinical dysfunction. Treatments which correct the pathomechanics have a favorable effect on pain and joint function [9].

1.3.2 Impairments in Muscle Function

Muscle function in the lower extremity, including weakness, altered muscle activation patterns, and proprioceptive deficits, is commonly found in association with knee OA. Improvement of muscle strength is a key component of conservative management of knee OA and has been found to be effective in symptom reduction [10]. Whether exercise influences disease development and potentially stalls progression needs more study.

1.3.3 OA and Knee Injury

A 22-year prospective study of Finnish subjects [11] researched the association of new cases of OA over time, diagnosed by physicians using information on disease histories, symptoms, and standardized clinical examinations. The risk of developing knee OA was strongly associated with BMI (kg/m^2) (adjusted for age, sex, and other covariates), as well as the heaviest category of physical stress at work (compared with the lightest category), and past knee injury.

A recent meta-analysis pooling 24 observational studies (20,997 subjects) was performed [12]. This analysis also included seven cohort studies, five cross-sectional studies, and 12 case–control studies. The conclusion was that history of knee injury is a major risk factor for the development of knee OA irrespective of study design and definition of knee injury.

1.3.4 Sex

Knee OA has a strong female sex preponderance. Women develop more knee OA than men, based on the rate of knee arthroplasty surgery. Approximately 3 million women and 1.7 million men had TKA in the USA. Obesity is a stronger risk factor for knee OA in women than in men. Some of the reasons for this are speculated to be the following: women lose knee articular cartilage at a faster rate than men, female human articular chondrocytes may function better when estrogen is available, male human articular chondrocytes are more responsive to vitamin D metabolites than female cells, vitamin D receptors and mRNA for inflammatory cytokines are differentially expressed in degenerated cartilage in a sex-specific fashion, and subchondral bone osteoblasts exhibit sex-specific responses to estrogen [13].

Independent of the effects of obesity, altered metabolism is related to knee OA, and these relations differ for men and women. A recent review of articles discussing OA and the metabolic syndrome outlines factors suggesting that the etiology of OA is different in males than females at virtually every level: epidemiologic, radiographic, circulating biomarker, hormonal, and cellular levels [14].

1.3.5 Heavy Physical Work

Of note vibration, repetitive movement, and long hours of kneeling and squatting, standing, and solitary standing are associated with an increased risk of development of OA [15].

1.3.6 Obesity

Increased awareness of obesity's frequent relationship to metabolic and inflammatory activities has made researchers rethink the role of obesity and OA. Pound for pound, not all obesities are equivalent to the development of knee osteoarthritis; development appears to be strongly related to the coexistence of disordered glucose and lipid metabolism. Cytokines associated with adipose tissue, including leptin, adiponectin, and resistin, may influence osteoarthritis through direct joint degradation or control of local inflammatory processes [16]. Metabolic risk factors including obesity, hypertension, dyslipidemia, and impaired glucose tolerance raise not only the risk of occurrence of OA but also its progression. This risk rises with the increasing number of metabolic risk factors present [17].

Conclusion

1. There is no universal definition of arthritis. Improved clarity in defining the arthritis and its progression would help clinicians improve outcome metrics and thus clinical care. A working definition may differ between the clinician and the researcher.
2. The risk factors with the most frequent association with knee OA are age, obesity, female sex, prior joint trauma including repetitive workload, and metabolic syndrome.
3. The etiology of this disease and factors associated with progression are continuously refined by researchers and clinicians alike.

Acknowledgments We would like to acknowledge the contributions of Cris Hansen and for her collaboration and editorial assistance on this manuscript.

References

1. Lawrence RC, Felson DT, Helmick CG, et al. Estimates of the prevalence of arthritis and other rheumatic conditions in the United States. Part II. Arthritis Rheum. 2008;58(1):26–35.
2. Kellgren JH, Lawrence JS. Radiological assessment of osteo-arthrosis. Ann Rheum Dis. 1957;16(4): 494–502.
3. Braun HJ, Gold GE. Diagnosis of osteoarthritis: imaging. Bone. 2012;51(2):278–88.
4. Wu CW, Morrell MR, Heinze E, et al. Validation of American College of Rheumatology classification criteria for knee osteoarthritis using arthroscopically defined cartilage damage scores. Semin Arthritis Rheum. 2005;35(3):197–201.
5. van Spil WE, DeGroot J, Lems WF, Oostveen JCM, Lafeber FPJG. Serum and urinary biochemical markers for knee and hip-osteoarthritis: a systematic review applying the consensus BIPED criteria. Osteoarthritis Cartilage. 2010;18(5):605–12.
6. Lotz M, Martel-Pelletier J, Christiansen C, et al. Value of biomarkers in osteoarthritis: current status and perspectives. Ann Rheum Dis. 2013;72(11): 1756–63.
7. Sheehy L, Culham E, McLean L, et al. Validity and sensitivity to change of three scales for the radiographic assessment of knee osteoarthritis using images from the Multicenter Osteoarthritis Study (MOST). Osteoarthritis Cartilage. 2015;23(9): 1491–8.
8. Kraus VB, Blanco FJ, Englund M, et al. OARSI clinical trials recommendations: soluble biomarker assessments in clinical trials in osteoarthritis. Osteoarthritis Cartilage. 2015;23(5):686–97.
9. Felson DT. Osteoarthritis as a disease of mechanics. Osteoarthritis Cartilage. 2013;21(1):10–5.
10. Bennell KL, Wrigley TV, Hunt MA, Lim BW, Hinman RS. Update on the role of muscle in the genesis and management of knee osteoarthritis. Rheum Dis Clin North Am. 2013;39(1):145–76.
11. Toivanen AT, Heliovaara M, Impivaara O, et al. Obesity, physically demanding work and traumatic knee injury are major risk factors for knee osteoarthritis–a population-based study with a follow-up of 22 years. Rheumatology (Oxford). 2010;49(2):308–14.
12. McWilliams DF, Leeb BF, Muthuri SG, Doherty M, Zhang W. Occupational risk factors for osteoarthritis of the knee: a meta-analysis. Osteoarthritis Cartilage. 2011;19(7):829–39.
13. Boyan BD, Tosi L, Coutts R, et al. Sex differences in osteoarthritis of the knee. J Am Acad Orthop Surg. 2012;20(10):668–9.
14. Huffman KM, Kraus WE. Osteoarthritis and the metabolic syndrome: more evidence that the etiology of OA is different in men and women. Osteoarthritis Cartilage. 2012;20(7):603–4.
15. Yucesoy B, Charles LE, Baker B, Burchfiel CM. Occupational and genetic risk factors for osteoarthritis: a review. Work. 2015;50(2):261–73.
16. Sowers MR, Karvonen-Gutierrez CA. The evolving role of obesity in knee osteoarthritis. Curr Opin Rheumatol. 2010;22(5):533–7.
17. Yoshimura N, Muraki S, Oka H, et al. Accumulation of metabolic risk factors such as overweight, hypertension, dyslipidaemia, and impaired glucose tolerance raises the risk of occurrence and progression of knee osteoarthritis: a 3-year follow-up of the ROAD study. Osteoarthritis Cartilage. 2012;20(11):1217–26.
18. Altman RD, Hochberg M, Murphy Jr WA, Wolfe F, Lequesne M. Atlas of individual radiographic features in osteoarthritis. Osteoarthritis Cartilage. 1995; 3(Suppl A):3–70.
19. Kornaat PR, Ceulemans RY, Kroon HM, et al. MRI assessment of knee osteoarthritis: Knee Osteoarthritis

Scoring System (KOSS)–inter-observer and intra-observer reproducibility of a compartment-based scoring system. Skeletal Radiol. 2005;34(2):95–102.

20. Peterfy CG, Guermazi A, Zaim S, et al. Whole-Organ Magnetic Resonance Imaging Score (WORMS) of the knee in osteoarthritis. Osteoarthritis Cartilage. 2004; 12(3):177–90.

21. Hunter DJ, Lo GH, Gale D, Grainger AJ, Guermazi A, Conaghan PG. The reliability of a new scoring system for knee osteoarthritis MRI and the validity of bone marrow lesion assessment: BLOKS (Boston Leeds Osteoarthritis Knee Score). Ann Rheum Dis. 2008;67(2):206–11.

22. Andriacchi TP, Favre J, Erhart-Hledik JC, Chu CR. A systems view of risk factors for knee osteoarthritis reveals insights into the pathogenesis of the disease. Ann Biomed Eng. 2015;43(2):376–87.

23. Evangelou E, Valdes AM, Kerkhof HJ, et al. Meta-analysis of genome-wide association studies confirms a susceptibility locus for knee osteoarthritis on chromosome 7q22. Ann Rheum Dis. 2011;70(2):349–55.

24. Kerkhof HJ, Bierma-Zeinstra SM, Arden NK, et al. Prediction model for knee osteoarthritis incidence, including clinical, genetic and biochemical risk factors. Ann Rheum Dis. 2014;73(12):2116–21.

25. Lo GH, Driban JB, Kriska AM, et al. Habitual running any time in life is not detrimental and may be protective of symptomatic knee osteoarthritis. Data from the Osteoarthritis Initiative. American College of Rheumatology annual meeting, Boston, 2014.

26. Sanghi D, Mishra A, Sharma AC, et al. Elucidation of dietary risk factors in osteoarthritis knee–a case–control study. J Am Coll Nutr. 2015;34(1):15–20.

27. Apold H, Meyer HE, Nordsletten L, Furnes O, Baste V, Flugsrud GB. Risk factors for knee replacement due to primary osteoarthritis, a population based, prospective cohort study of 315,495 individuals. BMC Musculoskelet Disord. 2014;15:217.

28. Fanelli GC, Sousa PL, Edson CJ. Long-term followup of surgically treated knee dislocations: Stability restored, but arthritis is common. Clin Orthop Relat Res. 2014;472(9):2712–7.

29. Logerstedt DS, Zeni Jr J, Snyder-Mackler L. Sex differences in patients with different stages of knee osteoarthritis. Arch Phys Med Rehabil. 2014;95(12): 2376–81.

30. Silverwood V, Blagojevic-Bucknall M, Jinks C, Jordan JL, Protheroe J, Jordan KP. Current evidence on risk factors for knee osteoarthritis in older adults: a systematic review and meta-analysis. Osteoarthritis Cartilage. 2015;23(4):507–15.

31. Chundru R, Baum T, Nardo L, et al. Focal knee lesions in knee pairs of asymptomatic and symptomatic subjects with OA risk factors–data from the osteoarthritis initiative. Eur J Radiol. 2013;82(8):e367–73.

32. Jungmann PM, Kraus MS, Alizai H, et al. Association of metabolic risk factors with cartilage degradation assessed by T2 relaxation time at the knee: data from the osteoarthritis initiative. Arthritis Care Res (Hoboken). 2013;65(12):1942–50.

33. Martin KR, Kuh D, Harris TB, Guralnik JM, Coggon D, Wills AK. Body mass index, occupational activity, and leisure-time physical activity: an exploration of risk factors and modifiers for knee osteoarthritis in the 1946 British birth cohort. BMC Musculoskelet Disord. 2013;14:219.

34. Prieto-Alhambra D, Judge A, Javaid MK, Cooper C, Diez-Perez A, Arden NK. Incidence and risk factors for clinically diagnosed knee, hip and hand osteoarthritis: influences of age, gender and osteoarthritis affecting other joints. Ann Rheum Dis. 2014;73(9): 1659–64.

35. Hansen P, English M, Willick SE. Does running cause osteoarthritis in the hip or knee? PM R. 2012;4(5 Suppl):S117–21.

36. Palmer KT. Occupational activities and osteoarthritis of the knee. Br Med Bull. 2012;102:147–70.

37. Sridhar MS, Jarrett CD, Xerogeanes JW, Labib SA. Obesity and symptomatic osteoarthritis of the knee. J Bone Joint Surg Br. 2012;94(4):433–40.

38. Chaganti RK, Lane NE. Risk factors for incident osteoarthritis of the hip and knee. Curr Rev Musculoskelet Med. 2011;4(3):99–104.

39. Hovis KK, Stehling C, Souza RB, et al. Physical activity is associated with magnetic resonance imaging-based knee cartilage T2 measurements in asymptomatic subjects with and those without osteoarthritis risk factors. Arthritis Rheum. 2011;63(8): 2248–56.

40. Jones G, Schultz MG, Dore D. Physical activity and osteoarthritis of the knee: can MRI scans shed more light on this issue? Phys Sportsmed. 2011;39(3): 55–61.

41. Molloy MG, Molloy CB. Contact sport and osteoarthritis. Br J Sports Med. 2011;45(4):275–7.

42. Muthuri SG, McWilliams DF, Doherty M, Zhang W. History of knee injuries and knee osteoarthritis: a meta-analysis of observational studies. Osteoarthritis Cartilage. 2011;19(11):1286–93.

43. Muthuri SG, Hui M, Doherty M, Zhang W. What if we prevent obesity? Risk reduction in knee osteoarthritis estimated through a meta-analysis of observational studies. Arthritis Care Res (Hoboken). 2011;63(7):982–90.

44. Papavasiliou KA, Kenanidis EI, Potoupnis ME, Kapetanou A, Sayegh FE. Participation in athletic activities may be associated with later development of hip and knee osteoarthritis. Phys Sportsmed. 2011; 39(4):51–9.

45. Segal NA, Glass NA. Is quadriceps muscle weakness a risk factor for incident or progressive knee osteoarthritis? Phys Sportsmed. 2011;39(4):44–50.

46. Valdes AM, Spector TD. Genetic epidemiology of hip and knee osteoarthritis. Nat Rev Rheumatol. 2011; 7(1):23–32.

47. Yusuf E, Bijsterbosch J, Slagboom PE, Rosendaal FR, Huizinga TW, Kloppenburg M. Body mass index and alignment and their interaction as risk factors for progression of knees with radiographic signs of osteoarthritis. Osteoarthritis Cartilage. 2011;19(9):1117–22.

48. Klussmann A, Gebhardt H, Nubling M, et al. Individual and occupational risk factors for knee osteoarthritis: results of a case–control study in Germany. Arthritis Res Ther. 2010;12(3):R88.

49. Stehling C, Lane NE, Nevitt MC, Lynch J, McCulloch CE, Link TM. Subjects with higher physical activity levels have more severe focal knee lesions diagnosed with 3T MRI: analysis of a non-symptomatic cohort of the osteoarthritis initiative. Osteoarthritis Cartilage. 2010;18(6):776–86.

50. Blagojevic M, Jinks C, Jeffery A, Jordan KP. Risk factors for onset of osteoarthritis of the knee in older adults: a systematic review and meta-analysis. Osteoarthritis Cartilage. 2010;18(1):24–33.

Nonoperative Treatment Options for Knee Osteoarthritis

2

David A. Parker and Corey Scholes

Contents

D.A. Parker, FRACS (✉)
North Shore Knee Clinic, Sydney, NSW, Australia

Sydney Orthopaedic Research Institute,
Chatswood, NSW, Australia
e-mail: dparker@sydneyortho.com.au

C. Scholes, PhD
Sydney Orthopaedic Research Institute,
Chatswood, NSW, Australia

2.1 Introduction and Scope

This chapter provides a compilation of the latest knowledge regarding nonoperative treatment of knee osteoarthritis. The aim is to provide an accessible reference for clinicians to establish a coordinated and effective management plan with maximum patient involvement. It is hoped that this reference can provide clear guidance in the selection of known treatment options and provide useful guidelines for both initial counselling and subsequent active management of the disease.

Currently, both clinicians and patients are bombarded with information available on the Internet and popular media regarding "miracle cures" and "cutting edge therapies" for the treatment of knee osteoarthritis. The top ten search results from google.com.au and facebook.com reveal a spectrum of quality with regard to available information (Fig. 2.1). Overall, the information from Google included a mixture of credible, useful information, as well as some outdated information. However, a considerable amount of results would be considered as misinformation combined with sponsored content, which can be difficult for lay readers to discern the inherent bias.

To address the volume of potentially misleading information available to both clinicians and patients, this chapter has been compiled from guidelines released by authoritative sources and updated with a comprehensive literature search of updated information, with emphasis on the

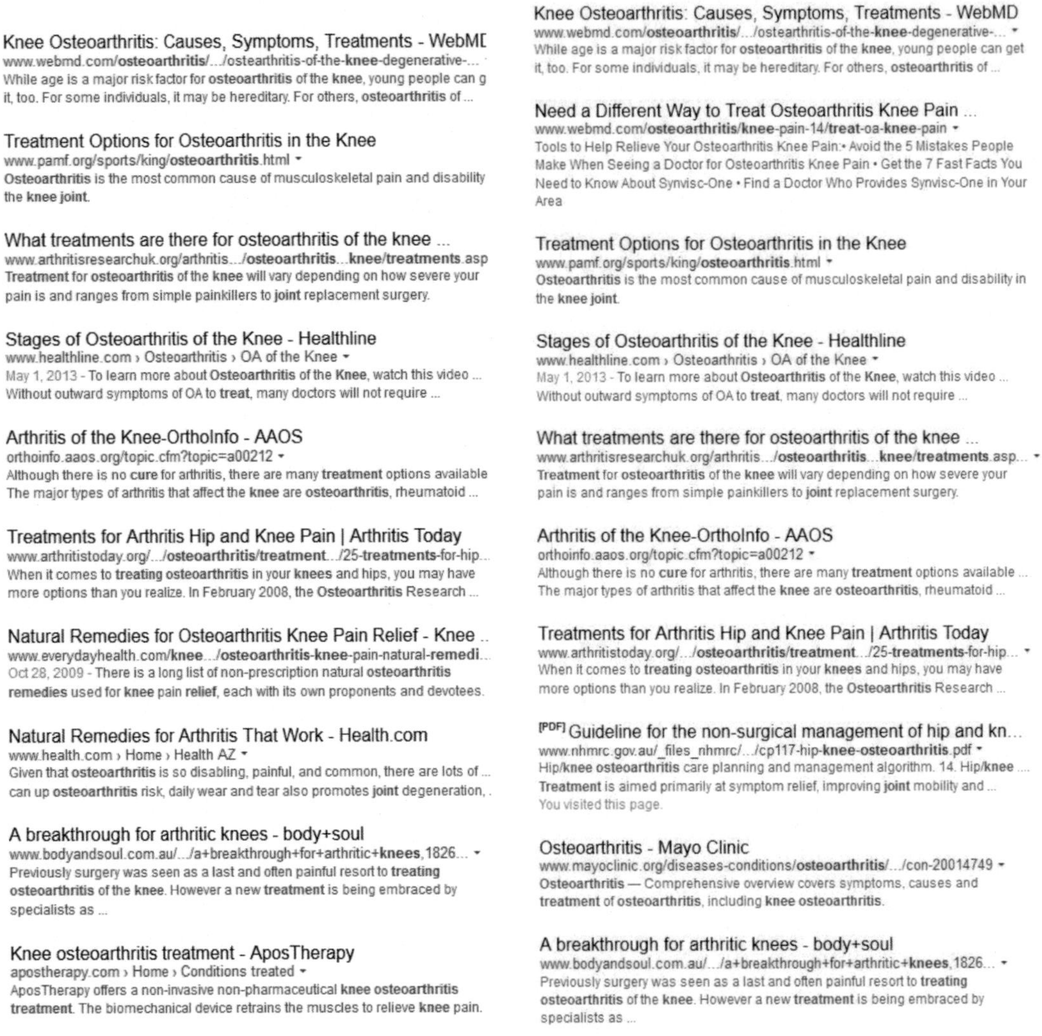

Knee Osteoarthritis: Causes, Symptoms, Treatments - WebMD
www.webmd.com/**osteoarthritis**/.../ostearthritis-of-the-**knee**-degenerative-...
While age is a major risk factor for **osteoarthritis** of the knee, young people can g
it, too. For some individuals, it may be hereditary. For others, **osteoarthritis** of ...

Treatment Options for Osteoarthritis in the Knee
www.pamf.org/sports/king/**osteoarthritis**.html
Osteoarthritis is the most common cause of musculoskeletal pain and disability
the **knee joint**.

What treatments are there for osteoarthritis of the knee ...
www.arthritisresearchuk.org/arthritis.../**osteoarthritis**...**knee**/treatments.asp
Treatment for **osteoarthritis** of the **knee** will vary depending on how severe your
pain is and ranges from simple painkillers to **joint** replacement surgery.

Stages of Osteoarthritis of the Knee - Healthline
www.healthline.com › Osteoarthritis › OA of the Knee
May 1, 2013 - To learn more about **Osteoarthritis** of the **Knee**, watch this video ...
Without outward symptoms of OA to **treat**, many doctors will not require ...

Arthritis of the Knee-OrthoInfo - AAOS
orthoinfo.aaos.org/topic.cfm?topic=a00212
Although there is no **cure** for arthritis, there are many **treatment** options available
The major types of arthritis that affect the **knee** are **osteoarthritis**, rheumatoid ...

Treatments for Arthritis Hip and Knee Pain | Arthritis Today
www.arthritistoday.org/.../**osteoarthritis**/treatment.../25-**treatments**-for-hip...
When it comes to **treating osteoarthritis** in your **knees** and hips, you may have
more options than you realize. In February 2008, the **Osteoarthritis** Research ...

Natural Remedies for Osteoarthritis Knee Pain Relief - Knee ..
www.everydayhealth.com/**knee**.../**osteoarthritis**-**knee**-pain-natural-**remedi**...
Oct 28, 2009 - There is a long list of non-prescription natural **osteoarthritis**
remedies used for **knee** pain **relief**, each with its own proponents and devotees.

Natural Remedies for Arthritis That Work - Health.com
www.health.com › Home › Health AZ
Given that **osteoarthritis** is so disabling, painful, and common, there are lots of ...
can up **osteoarthritis** risk, daily wear and tear also promotes **joint** degeneration, .

A breakthrough for arthritic knees - body+soul
www.bodyandsoul.com.au/.../a+breakthrough+for+arthritic+**knees**,1826...
Previously surgery was seen as a last and often painful resort to **treating**
osteoarthritis of the **knee**. However a new **treatment** is being embraced by
specialists as ...

Knee osteoarthritis treatment - AposTherapy
apostherapy.com › Home › Conditions treated
AposTherapy offers a non-invasive non-pharmaceutical **knee osteoarthritis**
treatment. The biomechanical device retrains the muscles to relieve **knee** pain.

Knee Osteoarthritis: Causes, Symptoms, Treatments - WebMD
www.webmd.com/**osteoarthritis**/.../ostearthritis-of-the-**knee**-degenerative-...
While age is a major risk factor for **osteoarthritis** of the knee, young people can get
it, too. For some individuals, it may be hereditary. For others, **osteoarthritis** of ...

Need a Different Way to Treat Osteoarthritis Knee Pain ...
www.webmd.com/**osteoarthritis**/**knee**-pain-14/**treat**-oa-**knee**-pain
Tools to Help Relieve Your Osteoarthritis Knee Pain. • Avoid the 5 Mistakes People
Make When Seeing a Doctor for Osteoarthritis Knee Pain • Get the 7 Fast Facts You
Need to Know About Synvisc-One • Find a Doctor Who Provides Synvisc-One in Your
Area

Treatment Options for Osteoarthritis in the Knee
www.pamf.org/sports/king/**osteoarthritis**.html
Osteoarthritis is the most common cause of musculoskeletal pain and disability in
the **knee joint**.

Stages of Osteoarthritis of the Knee - Healthline
www.healthline.com › Osteoarthritis › OA of the Knee
May 1, 2013 - To learn more about **Osteoarthritis** of the **Knee**, watch this video ...
Without outward symptoms of OA to **treat**, many doctors will not require ...

What treatments are there for osteoarthritis of the knee ...
www.arthritisresearchuk.org/arthritis.../**osteoarthritis**...**knee**/treatments.asp...
Treatment for **osteoarthritis** of the **knee** will vary depending on how severe your
pain is and ranges from simple painkillers to **joint** replacement surgery.

Arthritis of the Knee-OrthoInfo - AAOS
orthoinfo.aaos.org/topic.cfm?topic=a00212
Although there is no **cure** for arthritis, there are many **treatment** options available ...
The major types of arthritis that affect the **knee** are **osteoarthritis**, rheumatoid ...

Treatments for Arthritis Hip and Knee Pain | Arthritis Today
www.arthritistoday.org/.../**osteoarthritis**/treatment.../25-**treatments**-for-hip...
When it comes to **treating osteoarthritis** in your **knees** and hips, you may have
more options than you realize. In February 2008, the **Osteoarthritis** Research ...

[PDF] Guideline for the non-surgical management of hip and kn...
www.nhmrc.gov.au/_files_nhmrc/.../cp117-hip-**knee**-**osteoarthritis**.pdf
Hip/**knee osteoarthritis** care planning and management algorithm. 14. Hip/**knee** ...
Treatment is aimed primarily at symptom relief, improving **joint** mobility and ...
You visited this page.

Osteoarthritis - Mayo Clinic
www.mayoclinic.org/diseases-conditions/**osteoarthritis**/.../con-20014749
Osteoarthritis — Comprehensive overview covers symptoms, causes and
treatment of osteoarthritis, including **knee osteoarthritis**.

A breakthrough for arthritic knees - body+soul
www.bodyandsoul.com.au/.../a+breakthrough+for+arthritic+**knees**,1826...
Previously surgery was seen as a last and often painful resort to **treating**
osteoarthritis of the **knee**. However a new **treatment** is being embraced by
specialists as ...

Fig. 2.1 First page of search results from google.com.au using the terms "treatments for knee osteoarthritis"

highest quality systematic reviews and meta-analyses of current evidence.

2.2 Authoritative Recommendations

The Osteoarthritis Research Society International (OARSI) recently released an evidence-based summary of recommended treatment options for knee osteoarthritis [1]. The options recommended are summarised in Fig. 2.2 and comprise a set of *core treatments*, suggested for the management of all types of osteoarthritis in all individuals, as well as treatment options specific to knee OA for individuals with and without serious comorbidities.

Similarly, the American Academy of Orthopaedic Surgeons (AAOS) has also released a 2nd edition of their clinical practice guidelines for first-line treatment of knee OA [2]. These recommendations are summarised in Table 2.1 and address a number of options not covered in the OARSI recommendations. However, the AAOS clinical practice guidelines are older (2013), and updated information has since become available for a number of recommendations.

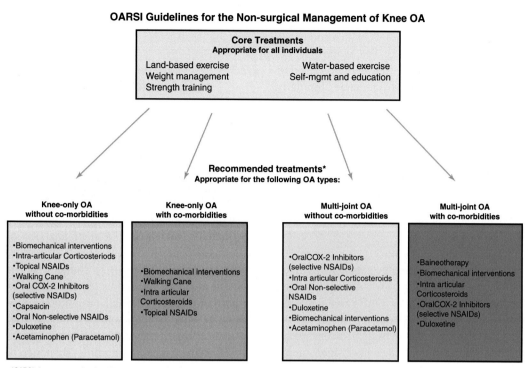

Fig. 2.2 OARSI guidelines for non-surgical management of knee OA [1]

Table 2.1 Summary of AAOS clinical practice guidelines for non-operative treatment of knee OA [2]

Treatment	Recommendation	Strength	Updated information
1. Self-management; strengthening; low-impact aerobic exercise; neuromuscular education; physical activity	Recommended	Strong	Yes
2. Weight loss BMI > 25	Suggested	Moderate	No change
3. (a) Acupuncture	Unable to recommend	Inconclusive	None available
(b) Physical agents (electrotherapy)	Unable to recommend	Inconclusive	No change
(c) Manual therapy	Unable to recommend	Inconclusive	Yes
4. Valgus-directing knee brace	Unable to recommend	Inconclusive	Yes
5. Lateral wedge insoles	Unable to recommend	Moderate	Yes
6. Glucosamine or chondroitin	Cannot be recommend	Strong	Yes
7. (a) NSAIDS or tramadol	Recommended	Strong	No change
(b) Acetaminophen	Unable to recommend	Inconclusive	Yes
8. Intra-articular corticosteroids	Unable to recommend	Inconclusive	Yes
9. Hyaluronic Acid	Cannot recommend	Strong	Yes

2.2.1 Core Treatments

2.2.1.1 Exercise

Exercise is any targeted, prescribed or organised activity where participation occurs with the aim of improving strength, endurance, range of motion or aerobic capacity [1]. Exercise to treat knee OA can be based on land or in water, and reductions in pain and improvements in function are well established. The OARSI guidelines are based on a systematic review and a meta-analysis of randomised controlled trials, with a good overall quality of the evidence. The average size of the effect for land-based exercise on pain reduction ranges from small to moderate. Similarly, water-based exercise also provides beneficial effects on pain and function, although the expected size of the effect has yet to be established. A more recent systematic review [3] of high-quality evidence reported that land-based exercise provided a moderate short-term (up to 6 months post-treatment) reduction in pain and improved physical function.

2.2.1.2 Strength Training

Exercise that specifically targets the ability of muscles to generate force, known as strength training, has been singled out in the OARSI recommendations as a key modality to reduce pain and improve physical function for knee OA. In particular, targeting the quadriceps and other lower-limb muscle groups should be considered as a key treatment option. Strength training can take a variety of forms, but recent evidence has been based on exercises conducted on land in group or individual sessions, and training combined with mobilisation is considered most effective.

2.2.1.3 Weight Loss

Being overweight or obese is a significant risk factor for knee osteoarthritis in older adults [4, 5]. Weight loss is particularly important for individuals diagnosed with knee OA who are also considered overweight or obese. Although a programme involving diet modification with exercise is considered most effective, a moderate reduction in weight (5 % of bodyweight) over a 20-week period provides small to moderate reductions in pain and improves physical function [1]. These recommendations are based on good-quality evidence from a systematic review and meta-analysis of randomised controlled trials. A more recent systematic review [6] suggests that weight reduction with combined diet modification and exercise is effective for pain relief and functional improvements even in elderly individuals (70+years). Involvement of a dietitian

and/or an exercise physiologist may be helpful in achieving these goals.

2.2.1.4 Self-Management and Education Programmes

Self-management programmes are distinct from patient education as they encourage people diagnosed with chronic disease to actively participate in the treatment of their condition [7]. The OARSI guidelines [1] suggest that self-management and education programmes can provide a small amount of pain reduction based on good-quality evidence stemming from a systematic review and a meta-analysis of randomised controlled trials. However, a more recent systematic review [7] found that the available evidence was of low to moderate quality but confirmed that such programmes provide no or small benefits up to 21 months after treatment. Importantly, this review reported that self-management programmes do not compare favourably to attention control methods or usual care.

2.2.1.5 Biomechanical Interventions

Treatment of knee OA should focus on the mechanical behaviour of the affected knee at any stage of disease progression but particularly at initial diagnosis in those with early signs [8]. Interventions designed to adjust knee and lower-limb loading during locomotion vary considerably. However, the OARSI guidelines focus on foot orthoses or shoe inserts or valgus knee braces. Foot orthoses alter the mechanical alignment of the lower leg by enhancing the valgus correction of the calcaneus, while braces apply an opposing valgus force to attenuate load on the medial knee compartment [9]. The proposed benefits of these interventions include pain reduction, reduced analgesic dosage, improved physical function, stiffness and potentially slowing disease progression. A more recent systematic review and meta-analysis [10] of valgus bracing reported a moderate to high effect on the knee adduction moment, which has been associated with disease progression [11], although the quality of current evidence remains fair.

2.2.2 Treatments Specifically for Knee Osteoarthritis

2.2.2.1 Intra-articular Injection of Corticosteroids

Corticosteroids mimic naturally occurring hormones that are anti-inflammatory in function. Common agents used to treat knee OA include betamethasone, methylprednisolone and triamcinolone which are injected directly into the joint space. The expected benefits of these injections are short-term pain relief, improved physical function and reduced joint inflammation. The current OARSI guidelines [1] suggest that corticosteroids are effective in providing short-term pain relief but are likely not appropriate for longer-term pain management. A more recent systematic review using network meta-analysis confirmed the effectiveness of corticosteroids in pain relief but reported a lack of effectiveness for improving joint function and stiffness. An earlier systematic review reported that the clinical response to injection may vary and can be predicted based on demographic and clinical factors [12].

2.2.2.2 Non-steroidal Anti-inflammatory Drugs (NSAIDs)

These medications have an anti-inflammatory effect and can be applied topically on the affected joint or taken orally. Oral NSAIDs are separated into Cox-2 inhibitors or non-selective options, and there is a risk of adverse events with extended use, despite moderate effects on pain. Cox-2 medications are felt to have a safer side effect profile than non-selective medications. Although the overall effect size of topical NSAIDs remains unknown, they are considered safer and better tolerated than oral NSAIDs. While oral NSAIDs are usually quite effective in pain management, their potential side effect profile makes them more suited to occasional rather than regular use, and caution should be employed in patients with any history of peptic ulceration and renal disease in particular.

2.2.2.3 Capsaicin

Capsaicin is a capsicum extract with anti-inflammatory properties which is applied topically. Although it has potential to reduce joint inflammation, reduce pain and increase function, based on good-quality evidence (systematic review and meta-analysis of randomised controlled trials), its effects range from small to moderate for reducing pain and improving function compared to placebo.

2.2.2.4 Duloxetine

Duloxetine is a serotonin-norepinephrine reuptake inhibitor and is usually prescribed as an antidepressant. Although there is fair evidence available based on systematic reviews and randomised trials, the size of its effect on knee pain remains unavailable; however, it has been reported to significantly decrease pain and improve physical function in knee OA.

2.2.2.5 Acetaminophen

Also known as paracetamol, this is commonly prescribed for a wide spectrum of pain, including knee OA. Good-quality evidence suggests that it has a small to moderate effect for pain and function, while a more recent review [12] suggests that its effects are small for pain relief. This is a medication than can be used regularly due to the relatively safe side effect profile and is probably more effective if used regularly.

2.3 Additional Treatment Options

2.3.1 Psychological Therapies

An individual's mental health is associated with the severity of their knee OA pain and risk of pain flares [13], with depression in particular associated with self-reported pain levels [14]. Psychological therapies have demonstrated efficacy in reducing pain, disability, depression and anxiety. Cognitive behavioural therapy is the most common approach reported in the literature and is typically delivered either in-person in group or individual sessions or via the Internet. Recent systematic reviews of low-quality evidence have reported small to moderate effects on pain using traditional therapy methods [15] or by Internet delivery [16] in adults experiencing chronic pain for reasons other than headache but not specific to knee OA. However, there is potential in the future for psychological therapies to provide some benefit to individuals experiencing pain related to knee OA with little risk of adverse side effects.

2.3.2 Chondroitin

Chondroitin is a nutritional supplement containing chondroitin sulphate which is normally found in articular cartilage, and its loss is potentially associated with the progression of osteoarthritis in the knee. Supplementing chondroitin orally is thought to possibly provide pain reduction and may modify the disease process. Recent systematic reviews are favourable for its ability to achieve these effects with one review of low-quality evidence [17] reporting an overall 10 % reduction in pain compared to placebo, while another review of moderate-quality evidence concluded that chondroitin significantly reduced cartilage loss in OA knees compared to placebo [18]. Although these results should probably be treated with caution, considering its non-invasive nature and low risk of negative side effects, chondroitin could be considered a treatment option, particularly for early stage knee osteoarthritis.

2.3.3 Glucosamine

Glucosamine is an aminosaccharide naturally occurring in the body and is a principal substrate in the synthesis of proteoglycan, a key component of articular cartilage. Glucosamine therapy is provided as a nutritional supplement available without prescription. A recent systematic review of low-quality evidence [18] suggested that glucosamine sulphate is moderately effective at reducing pain associated with knee OA, while a second recent review of moderate-quality evidence [19] also indicated a significant reduction of cartilage loss compared to placebo for glucosamine sulphate, but not for glucosamine

hydrochloride. Glucosamine sulphate provides a potential non-invasive treatment option, with a good safety profile for clinicians and patients to reduce pain and possibly slow the progression of cartilage loss and could be considered a possible option for early stage knee osteoarthritis treatment. As with chondroitin, although there are some studies showing positive results with glucosamine, the overall review of literature pertaining to these products would suggest that the evidence for clinical efficacy is modest, and therefore they cannot be strongly recommended for routine use.

2.3.4 Viscosupplementation

Refers to the intra-articular injection of hyaluronic acid, which is a main component of synovial fluid. Its proposed benefits include pain reduction, improved physical function and a low-risk of harm, with a particular emphasis on short-term improvement in pain post-injection. The current OARSI and AAOS guidelines are either unable to recommend viscosupplementation as a treatment option or indicate uncertain appropriateness. However, recent systematic reviews [12, 20] of low- to moderate-quality evidence reported moderate to large effects on pain relief, although variability in the clinical response was identified as a limiting factor [20]. A more recent review [21] of meta-analyses with low- to high-quality studies reported that intra-articular injection of hyaluronic acid improved function for up 6 months after treatment and was a viable option for patients with early stage knee osteoarthritis. Many of these more favourable studies should be interpreted with caution as they have been sponsored studies, and when the non-independent studies are excluded, the benefit would seem questionable.

2.3.5 Autologous Concentrated Plasma (ACP) or Platelet-Rich Plasma (PRP)

Platelet-derived growth factors regulate some processes in tissue repair. Currently, these factors are derived from a patient's own blood sample and injected directly into the joint space after appropriate preparation. The scientific literature presently suffers from a lack of consensus on the clinical efficacy of these treatments. One systematic review [22] of eight articles with low- to moderate-quality evidence concluded that PRP efficacy remains uncertain. However, a systematic review and meta-analysis [23] of moderate-quality evidence indicated that PRP provides effective pain relief at least 6 months post-injection. In addition, a review of three meta-analyses of low- to high-quality evidence [24] found that PRP injections improved pain and function as early as 2 months after treatment with peak improvement at 6 months, with symptomatic relief for up to 12months. These authors concluded that particularly those with mild to moderate osteoarthritic changes in the knee should consider this as a treatment option.

2.3.6 Gait Modification

The first-line approaches for early knee osteoarthritis should target the loading patterns around the knee during common daily activities [8]. Although biomechanical interventions should be an important part of OA treatment, the current OARSI guidelines only recommend the use of foot orthoses or valgus braces. However, the loads imposed on the knee during walking can also vary with different walking strategies. One systematic review [25] of low- to moderate-quality evidence suggested that the knee adduction moment, a key loading parameter in the progression of knee OA, can be reduced by increasing a person's step width or hip internal rotation, increasing their trunk lean or by encouraging an inward (medial) knee thrust or inward foot weight transfer.

A more recent review [26] of low- to moderate-quality evidence also reported that reductions in knee adduction moment could be achieved by altering foot progression angle (toe-in or toe-out), shortening stride length, leaning the trunk to one side or encouraging an inward thrust of the knee during weight bearing. Gait retraining offers

a low-cost and low-risk option for intervention in knee osteoarthritis; however, modifications that are suitable for each individual may take time to identify due to the natural variation of gait patterns and will require a concerted effort on the part of both clinician and patient. Clinicians and patients should also be prepared to manage the potential for gait modification to shift load to other joints, particularly in patients with joints other than the knee affected by osteoarthritis or significant comorbidities.

2.3.7 Stem Cell Therapy

Stem cells are theoretically capable of differentiating into a range of specialised cells, with particular emphasis in therapeutic applications for osteoarthritis for their capacity to regenerate cartilage. For stem cell therapy, cells can be derived from mesenchyme (bone marrow), adipose tissue, the patient's own synovium or allogenic umbilical cord material. Unfortunately, despite its theoretical potential, the evidence of clinical efficacy remains weak, with a recent clinical review [27] of low- to moderate-quality evidence highlighting the lack of in vivo data for these therapies. At this time, stem cell therapy cannot be recommended as a viable treatment option for knee osteoarthritis, but is certainly an appropriate area for ongoing clinical research to better define the treatment and its role in OA.

2.4 Recommended Treatment Strategy for Knee OA

A limitation of the current guidelines and authoritative evidence is the lack of integration between treatment modalities and guidance for the clinician in regard to the optimal approach for any given patient. Although considerable amounts of research are required to address this gap with high-quality evidence, evidence-based recommendations have been released by the European Union League Against Rheumatism (EULAR) [28] for non-pharmacological management of knee OA, with a framework for applying many of

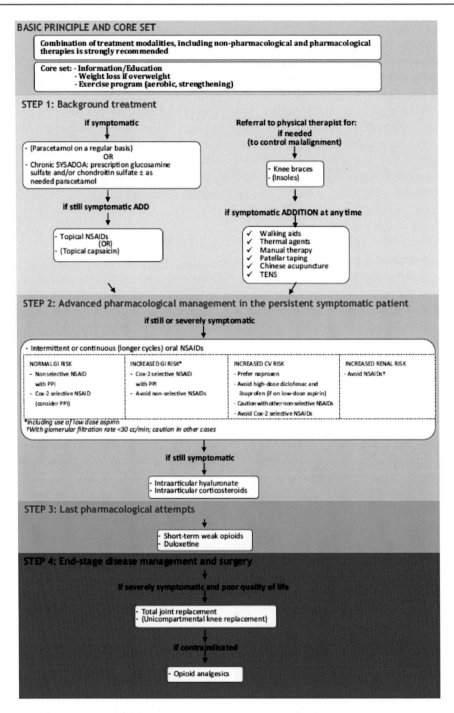

Fig. 2.3 Proposed treatment algorithm for knee osteoarthritis [29]

the treatment options covered in this chapter. Other recent attempts to develop treatment algorithms for knee OA have been presented (Fig. 2.3) [29]. A limitation of the model illustrated in Fig. 2.3 is its linear nature between diagnosis and disease progression to end-stage intervention. In the early stages of the disease, it is likely that the clinician and the patient may move through a

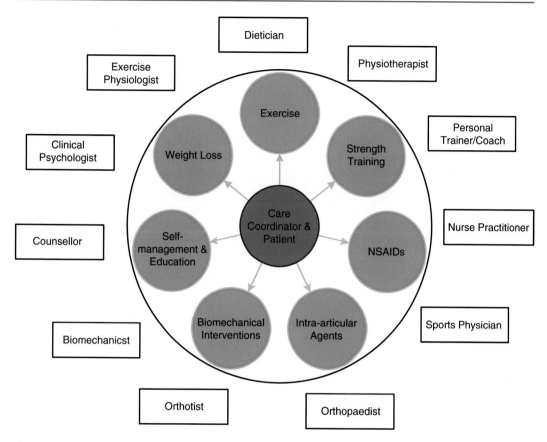

Fig. 2.4 Proposed model of coordinated care for non-operative treatment of knee osteoarthritis

range of modalities in a circular manner as the severity of pain and functional disability varies.

An ongoing difficulty that the clinician faces in managing OA non-operatively is initially convincing patients of the value of the multidisciplinary approach and subsequently providing a coordinated programme that ensures patients get the appropriate treatment from each of the modalities in a clear and well-managed fashion. For patients, this requires a clear explanation of the problem and the proposed solutions and sufficient education so that the treatment pathway and goals are clear to the patient. Written and Web-based resources can be provided for the patient and a clear timetable for treatment including regular assessments to evaluate progress and modify programs accordingly. A central coordinator such as a nurse practitioner who has a good relationship with the patient and can help coordinate treatment, advise and provide regular

feedback is central to the success of this type of program.

Therefore, based on the literature summarised in this chapter, a coordinated-care model is recommended with specialists engaged to apply specific treatment modalities where appropriate. A key emphasis of this approach is coordinated care and ongoing feedback from the patient regarding the care plan and effects of specific treatments with a close working relationship between the care coordinator, the patient and specialists (Fig. 2.4). The care coordinator should be an appropriately qualified health professional such as a nurse or general practitioner, and the key traits of a successful coordinator are a basic understanding of the mechanisms of each treatment option and an ability to establish and maintain an interpersonal relationship with the patient.

The care coordinator should be actively involved in determining the key treatment priorities with a thorough needs analysis, including assessment of symptoms and disability using standardised and validated instruments. From the patient clinical profile, a patient-specific model of care should be established in collaboration with the patient that targets the priority symptoms with the safest and least invasive modalities in the first instance, with focus on the core treatment options (Fig. 2.4). The care coordinator should aim to perform a thorough reassessment of the patient's condition at appropriate milestones, such as conclusion of supervised therapy. Positive feedback to the patient regarding the effectiveness of the program improves compliance and likelihood of sustaining ongoing improvement.

has also presented some recommendations for how patient care should be arranged in a coordinated manner with a close working relationship between a care coordinator and the patient, with a mix of specialists providing specific treatment input where appropriate. Although the recommendations for non-surgical management of knee osteoarthritis will continue to rapidly evolve, this chapter provides a basis for clinicians and patients to have an informed discussion on current treatment options for optimising non-surgical management of knee OA. This should always predate any discussion of surgical management and hopefully if applied effectively, will allow appropriate deferment of surgical management until absolutely necessary.

2.5   Summary and Conclusions

Historically knee osteoarthritis has been thought to have very limited treatment options, but clinicians and patients in the present day have many options to relieve symptoms and restore function reasonably quickly and safely. Many of the regularly promoted options have questionable clinical efficacy and safety, and it can be difficult to separate valid evidence from advertising to determine the most appropriate options with information publicly available, particularly through popular Web search engines. For this reason, this chapter has highlighted a series of core non-surgical treatment options based on the highest quality consensus recommendations from authoritative sources. In addition, a series of options have been identified that could provide viable treatments, with evidence of clinical efficacy that has been established since publication of the consensus recommendations. Given the limited surgical options, particularly for younger patients, establishing and maintaining optimal non-surgical treatment is critical for these patients and is an area that all health professionals managing these patients should be familiar with.

The onset and progression of knee osteoarthritis is a multifactorial and complex process, which can be targeted by a dynamic and adaptive mix of treatment options for symptom relief in the early stages of the disease. In light of this, this chapter

References

1. McAlindon TE, et al. OARSI guidelines for the non-surgical management of knee osteoarthritis. Osteoarthritis Cartilage. 2014;22(3):363–88.
2. Jevsevar DS. Treatment of osteoarthritis of the knee: evidence-based guideline, 2nd edition. J Am Acad Orthop Surg. 2013;21(9):571–6.
3. Fransen M, et al. Exercise for osteoarthritis of the knee. Cochrane Database Syst Rev. 2015;1:CD004376.
4. Silverwood V, et al. Current evidence on risk factors for knee osteoarthritis in older adults: a systematic review and meta-analysis. Osteoarthritis Cartilage. 2015;23(4):507–15.
5. Richmond SA, et al. Are joint injury, sport activity, physical activity, obesity, or occupational activities predictors for osteoarthritis? A systematic review. J Orthop Sports Phys Ther. 2013;43(8):515–B19.
6. Quintrec JL, et al. Physical exercise and weight loss for hip and knee osteoarthritis in very old patients: a systematic review of the literature. Open Rheumatol J. 2014;8:89–95.
7. Kroon FP, et al. Self-management education programmes for osteoarthritis. Cochrane Database Syst Rev. 2014;1:CD008963.
8. Arendt EA, Miller LE, Block JE. Early knee osteoarthritis management should first address mechanical joint overload. Orthop Rev (Pavia). 2014;6(1):5188.
9. Raja K, Dewan N. Efficacy of knee braces and foot orthoses in conservative management of knee osteoarthritis: a systematic review. Am J Phys Med Rehabil. 2011;90(3):247–62.
10. Moyer RF, et al. Biomechanical effects of valgus knee bracing: a systematic review and meta-analysis. Osteoarthritis Cartilage. 2015;23(2):178–88.
11. Chang AH, et al. External knee adduction and flexion moments during gait and medial tibiofemoral disease

progression in knee osteoarthritis. Osteoarthritis Cartilage. 2015;23(7):1099–106.

12. Bannuru RR, et al. Comparative effectiveness of pharmacologic interventions for knee osteoarthritis: a systematic review and network meta-analysis. Ann Intern Med. 2015;162(1):46–54.

13. Wise BL, et al. Psychological factors and their relation to osteoarthritis pain. Osteoarthritis Cartilage. 2010;18(7):883–7.

14. Phyomaung PP, et al. Are depression, anxiety and poor mental health risk factors for knee pain? A systematic review. BMC Musculoskelet Disord. 2014; 15:10.

15. Williams AC, Eccleston C, Morley S. Psychological therapies for the management of chronic pain (excluding headache) in adults. Cochrane Database Syst Rev. 2012;11:CD007407.

16. Eccleston C, et al. Psychological therapies (Internet-delivered) for the management of chronic pain in adults. Cochrane Database Syst Rev. 2014;2:CD010152.

17. Singh JA, et al. Chondroitin for osteoarthritis. Cochrane Database Syst Rev. 2015;1:CD005614.

18. Gallagher B, et al. Chondroprotection and the prevention of osteoarthritis progression of the knee: a systematic review of treatment agents. Am J Sports Med. 2015;43(3):734–44.

19. Percope de Andrade MA, Campos TV, Abreu-E-Silva GM. Supplementary methods in the nonsurgical treatment of osteoarthritis. Arthroscopy. 2015;31(4): 785–92.

20. Evaniew N, Simunovic N, Karlsson J. Cochrane in CORR(R): viscosupplementation for the treatment of osteoarthritis of the knee. Clin Orthop Relat Res. 2014;472(7):2028–34.

21. Campbell KA, et al. Is local viscosupplementation injection clinically superior to other therapies in the treatment of osteoarthritis of the knee: a systematic review of overlapping meta-analyses. Arthroscopy. 2015;31(10):2036–45.

22. Lai LP, et al. Use of platelet rich plasma in intra-articular knee injections for osteoarthritis: a systematic review. PM R. 2015;7(6):637–48.

23. Laudy AB, et al. Efficacy of platelet-rich plasma injections in osteoarthritis of the knee: a systematic review and meta-analysis. Br J Sports Med. 2015;49(10):657–72.

24. Campbell KA, et al. Does intra-articular platelet-rich plasma injection provide clinically superior outcomes compared with other therapies in the treatment of knee osteoarthritis? A systematic review of overlapping meta-analyses. Arthroscopy. 2015. Article in press.

25. Simic M, et al. Gait modification strategies for altering medial knee joint load: a systematic review. Arthritis Care Res (Hoboken). 2011;63(3):405–26.

26. Khalaj N, et al. Effect of exercise and gait retraining on knee adduction moment in people with knee osteoarthritis. Proc Inst Mech Eng H. 2014;228(2):190–9.

27. Wolfstadt JI, et al. Current concepts: the role of mesenchymal stem cells in the management of knee osteoarthritis. Sports Health. 2015;7(1):38–44.

28. Fernandes L, et al. EULAR recommendations for the non-pharmacological core management of hip and knee osteoarthritis. Ann Rheum Dis. 2013;72(7):1125–35.

29. Bruyere O, et al. An algorithm recommendation for the management of knee osteoarthritis in Europe and internationally: a report from a task force of the European Society for Clinical and Economic Aspects of Osteoporosis and Osteoarthritis (ESCEO). Semin Arthritis Rheum. 2014;44(3):253–63.

Part II

Surgical Management

Meniscus Surgery

3

Ashok Rajgopal and Attique Vasdev

Contents

3.1 Anatomy and Development of the Meniscus

The menisci (Fig. 3.1) are two crescent-shaped fibrocartilaginous structures that are found within each knee between the femoral condyles and the tibial plateau. Earlier, they were considered as functionless remnants of a leg muscle [1]. In 1942, Murray [2] stated that "when the knee joint is opened on the anterior aspect and the suspected cartilage appears normal, its removal can be undertaken with confidence if the diagnosis of a posterior tear has been arrived at clinically prior to the operation. A far too common error is shown in the incomplete removal of the injured meniscus."

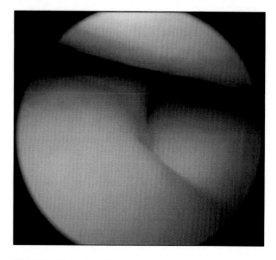

Fig. 3.1 Normal meniscus

A. Rajgopal, MS, Mch(Orth), FRCS (✉)
A. Vasdev, MS (Orth)
Medanta Bone and Joint Institute,
Medanta- the Medicity, Gurgaon, India
e-mail: a_rajgopal@hotmail.com

© ISAKOS 2016
D.A. Parker (ed.), *Management of Knee Osteoarthritis in the Younger, Active Patient:
An Evidence-Based Practical Guide for Clinicians*, DOI 10.1007/978-3-662-48530-9_3

The menisci enhance the stability of the knee joint by deepening and hence increasing the contact area between the femoral condyles and the tibial plateau. They help dissipate the contact hoop forces evenly across the articular surface. By virtue of the nerve endings in their anterior and posterior thirds, they contribute to the proprioception in the knee joint. The menisci also aid in lubrication in the knee joint [1, 2].

3.1.1   Embryology

In the developing embryo in the 28th–32nd day stage, the lower limb buds form opposite the lower lumbar and upper sacral segments. Gardner and O' Rahilly [3], Mc Dermot [4] and others provided detailed descriptions of the prenatal development of the knee joint. However, they largely described the embryonic development of the joint (i.e., prior to three gestational months) [5]. Thus, the intra-uterine development is divided into four stages:

1. Formation of the uniform interzone:
   The osteogenesis of the long bones starts from the 6th week onwards from primary ossification centres in the middle of the cartilaginous anlage of the long bones.
2. Formation of the three-layered interzone:
   At the end of the embryonic period (8 weeks, stage 23), the cells of the menisci are round and randomly arranged. The superficial cells begin to orient themselves parallel to the joint surface.
3. Meniscal cell differentiation:
   A layer of decreased cell density separates the menisci from the tibial plateaux. By 10 weeks, the densely celled menisci can be easily distinguished from a loose celled tissue peripherally which contains blood vessels.
4. Collagenous matrix formation inside the menisci:
   At 12 weeks, some blood vessels penetrate the peripheral third of both menisci. The orientation of collagen fibres becomes obvious at 14 weeks: it is parallel to the joint surface on the inner part of the menisci, and by 40 weeks, the vascularity of the entire meniscus is defined.

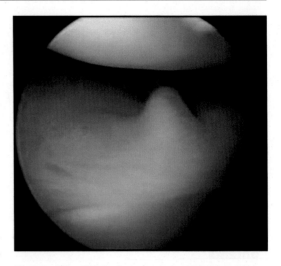

Fig. 3.2 Discoid lateral meniscus complete type

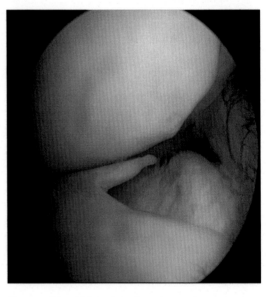

Fig. 3.3 Discoid lateral meniscus incomplete type

3.1.2   Discoid Meniscus

A congenital variant of the normal morphology of the meniscus is the discoid meniscus (Figs. 3.2 and 3.3). Smillie [6] suggested that this variation in structure is due to a failure of the foetal discoid form of meniscus to involute. He found in his series an incidence of around 6 %. A comprehensive study by Nathan and Cole [7] found 2.5 % of the menisci to be discoid. They are more common on the lateral side than the medial and rarely ever are found in both compartments. These can cause symptoms of snapping and popping in the knee in children, usually between the ages of 6 and 12 years.

The entity of discoid lateral meniscus was first reported by Young [8] in 1889. In a small percentage of these patients, there is no attachment of the posterior horn to the tibial plateau and instead a continuous Wrisberg ligament. This absent insertion may have implications for meniscal stability, although instability of clinical significance is uncommon.

Multiple classifications have been proposed, the most commonly used being the Watanabe et al. [9] system of 1978. They described three different types:

1. Complete, disk-shaped meniscus with a thin centre covering the tibial plateau
2. Incomplete, semilunar-shaped meniscus with partial tibial plateau coverage
3. Wrisberg-type, hypermobile meniscus resulting from deficient posterior tibial attachments

In 1998, Monllau et al. [10] identified a fourth type: the ring-shaped meniscus. Good et al. [11] proposed an interesting classification based on the discoid meniscal instability as anterior or posterior. In the vast majority of discoid menisci, the meniscus is simply an incidental finding on either MRI or arthroscopy and is asymptomatic.

3.1.3 Composition and Histology

Clarke and Ogden [12] are credited with the description of the postnatal development study of the human menisci, correlating anatomy and histology. The normal human meniscal tissue is composed of 72 % water, 22 % collagen, 0.8 % glycosaminoglycans and 0.12 % DNA [13]. Histologically, the menisci are fibrocartilaginous and are primarily composed of an interlacing network of collagen fibres interposed with cells, with an extracellular matrix of proteoglycans and glycoproteins. Type I collagen accounts for over 90 % of the meniscal collagen, the remainder consists of types II, II and IV [14]. Bullough

et al. [15] found that the principal orientation of the collagen fibre is circumferential, to withstand tension. They also found some radially oriented collagen fibres which were believed to act as "ties" holding the circumferential fibres together.

This arrangement provides good tensile strength and aids in evenly distributing forces across the articular surface [16]. The circumferential fibres absorb the compressive forces, whereas the radial fibres help prevent longitudinal splitting [17]. Disruption of the meniscal integrity leads to uneven loading of the joint cartilage, leading to early osteoarthritis [18]. Each meniscus is divided into three segments: anterior third, middle third (body) and posterior third. It is the outer 20–30 % which is vascular (red zone) and is supplied by the medial and lateral geniculate arteries, respectively. The inner two thirds of the menisci are relatively avascular (white zone). This distribution of blood supply determines the treatment of meniscal tears [19].

3.2 Role and Functions

Over the years, understanding the functions and roles of the menisci has changed dramatically, and since King's paper in 1936 [20], numerous studies have shown that the menisci play important roles. They have now been recognised as key primary stabilisers and weight transmitters in the knee and primarily distribute the contact forces across the tibiofemoral articulation, which is achieved through a combination of the material, geometry and attachments of the menisci. Fukubayashi and Kurosawa [21] examined the intra-articular contact areas using a casting method employing silicone rubber and found that the menisci combined occupied 70 % of the total contact area within the joint. Walker and Erkman [22] also used casting technique in their study and deduced that under no load, contact occurred primarily on the menisci, but that with loads of 150 kg and more, the menisci covered between 59 and 71 % of the joint contact surface area.

The medial meniscus is the larger of the two and covers about 50 % of the medial tibial plateau. The anterior third is attached to the medial tibial spine just (7 mm) anterior to the anterior cruciate ligament (ACL) insertion. The posterior third attaches anterior to the attachment of the posterior cruciate ligament (PCL). Medially, it is attached to the femoral condyle and tibial plateau by means of the coronary ligaments which form the deep portion of the medial collateral ligament [23]. The peripheral capsular attachment of the medial meniscus is continuous. This relative immobility of the medial meniscus renders it at a higher risk of injury when compared to the lateral meniscus [24, 25].

The lateral meniscus, which is the smaller of the two menisci, covers about 70 % of the lateral tibial plateau. The anterior third attaches anterior to the tibial spine sharing some fibres with the ACL. The posterior third is attached just posterior to the tibial spine [23]. The peripheral capsular attachment is interrupted by the popliteus hiatus through which passes the popliteus tendon. The meniscofemoral ligaments attach the posterior third of the lateral meniscus to the lateral margin of the posterior medial femoral condyle. The anterior part is called the ligament of Humphrey, and the posterior one is the ligament of Wrisberg. It is more mobile than the medial meniscus and may displace up to 1 cm, which may explain why meniscal injuries occur less frequently on the lateral side [24, 25].

The discoid meniscus (Figs. 3.2 and 3.3) is a developmental anomaly in which the meniscus is thickened and is disk shaped. Discoid medial menisci are very rare with a reported incidence of 0.06–0.3 % [26, 27] of the general population. Discoid lateral menisci are more common with a reported incidence of 1.4–15.5 % [28]. The Koreans and Japanese have a higher incidence (16 %) than the Caucasians (5 %) [29]. They are of three types: partial, complete and the Wrisberg type [30]. Partial and complete variants are determined by the amount of coverage of the tibial plateau. They have normal tibial attachments and are stable. The Wrisberg type has no posterior capsular and tibial attachment. The only attachment is the meniscofemoral ligament of Wrisberg. These are highly mobile and unstable but fortunately relatively uncommon.

3.3   Meniscal Tears

The incidence of meniscal tears is about 61/100,000 persons per year in the United States [31] and 60–70/100,000 persons in Europe [32]. This is a highly estimated figure as many tears are asymptomatic and a similarly high number is seen in degenerative knees. Meniscal tears are more common in males (male: female = 2.5:1 to 4:1). Anterior cruciate ligament injuries are associated with almost a third of meniscal tears, more commonly the lateral meniscus in the acute injury setting [33, 34].

Meniscal tears can occur as a result of acute events and also from chronic degeneration. Meniscal tears usually occur secondary to axial and rotational loads, and activities in which sudden stopping and turning movements occur lead to a majority of tears. Instability increases the risk of meniscal tear, and a significant number of tears occur with anterior cruciate ligament injuries. 32 % of meniscal tears happen during a sports injury, 39 % during activities of daily living such as squatting and 29 % do not have any identifiable cause/event [33].

Meniscal injuries are usually accompanied by sudden onset of pain in the involved knee followed by a delayed onset of swelling, and tenderness is usually present in the involved compartment. Mechanical symptoms such as locking, catching and giving way are frequently seen. Joint effusion is present and pain is felt on deep flexion or on squatting. Special tests include joint line tenderness and the McMurray and Apley grinding test. Joint line tenderness is the most sensitive test with a sensitivity of 74 %. A positive McMurray test with a palpable clunk is very specific for a meniscal tear (98 % specificity) but has a sensitivity of only 15 %. A positive Apley grinding test has a specificity of 70 % and sensitivity of 60 % [35–37]. Symptoms of associated ligament injuries may also manifest. Chronic degenerative tears present with episodes of mechanical symptoms. On top of the underlying pain of the degenerative process in the knee, the patient may complain of locking and/or catching of the knee. An injury or twisting episode is not necessary to produce these symptoms. Magnetic resonance imaging (MRI) is the investigation of

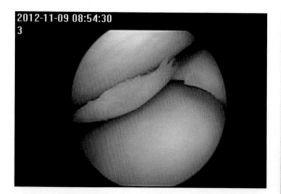

Fig. 3.4 Flap tear of medial meniscus

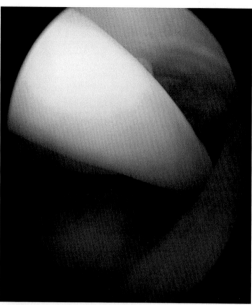

Fig. 3.6 Bucket handle displaced in notch

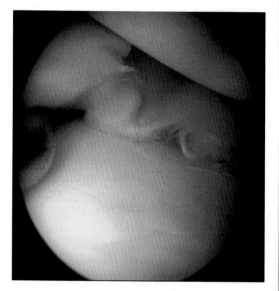

Fig. 3.5 Complex tear medial meniscus

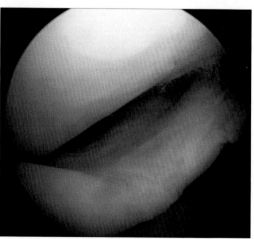

Fig. 3.7 Displaced bucket handle tear of medial meniscus

choice to detect meniscal tears. X-rays are often performed to rule out any osseous injury.

Meniscal tears are classified on the basis of tear location, tear pattern or by blood supply. On the basis of tear location, they are anterior horn tears, tears of the body, posterior horn tears and root avulsions. Tears classified on the basis of pattern of tear are flap tears (Fig. 3.4), radial tears, complex/degenerative tears (Fig. 3.5), longitudinal tears, bucket handle tears (Figs. 3.6, 3.7 and 3.8), parrot beak tears (Fig. 3.9) and horizontal tears [38]. Cooper et al. described a circumferential zone classification based on the blood supply of the meniscus. Zone 0 is the meniscosynovial junction, zone 1 is the outer third of the meniscus, zone 2 includes the middle third and zone 3 is the central third of the meniscus [39].

The International Society of Arthroscopy, Knee Surgery and Orthopaedic Sports Medicine (ISAKOS) formed a Meniscal Documentation Subcommittee in 2006 with the objective of developing a reliable, international meniscal evaluation and documentation system to facilitate outcomes assessment. In an interobserver

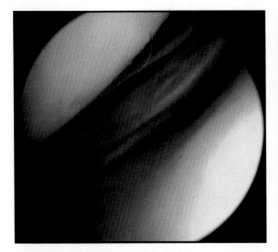

Fig. 3.8 Undisplaced bucket handle tear of medial meniscus

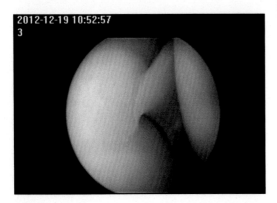

Fig. 3.9 Parrot beak tear of medial meniscus

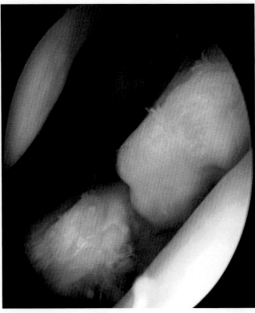

Fig. 3.10 Lateral meniscus root tear

reliability study, Anderson et al. [40] concluded that the ISAKOS classification of meniscal tears provided sufficient interobserver reliability for pooling of data from international clinical trials designed to evaluate the outcomes of treatment for meniscal tears.

Meniscal root tears (Fig. 3.10) differ distinctly from tears of the anterior or posterior horn of the meniscus. Meniscal roots are ligamentous attachments that help anchor the anterior and posterior horns of the meniscus to the tibial plateau. Root tears may or may not be associated with tears of the meniscus, and isolated root tears can occur with no meniscus tear itself. The meniscus is no longer anchored at the root attachment, leading to secondary extrusion. In this scenario, the meniscus will no longer perform its normal function of buffering the mechanical load imposed on the tibiofemoral joint, leading to tibiofemoral cartilage loss. In 2013 in a multicentre study, Guermazi et al. [41] concluded that isolated medial posterior meniscal root tear is associated with progressive medial tibiofemoral cartilage loss.

Based on tear morphology, LaPrade et al. [42] classified meniscal root tear patterns into the following:

Type 1: Partial stable root tears
Type 2: Complete radial tears within 9 mm of the bony root attachment (further subclassified into types 2A, 2B and 2C, located 0 to <3 mm, 3 to <6 mm and 6 to 9 mm from the root attachment, respectively)
Type 3: Bucket-handle tears with a complete root detachment
Type 4: Complex oblique tears with complete root detachments extending into the root attachment
Type 5: Bony avulsion fractures of the root attachments

Takahashi et al. in their study aimed to identify factors on routine pulse sequence MRI associated with cartilage degeneration observed on T1ρ relaxation mapping. They concluded that posterior root/horn radial tears in the medial meniscus are particularly important MRI findings associated with cartilage degeneration observed on T1ρ relaxation mapping. Morphological factors of the medial meniscus on MRI provide findings useful for screening early-stage osteoarthritis.

The importance of anatomical repair of meniscal root tears was emphasised by LaPrade et al. [43] in another study. They concluded that the non-anatomic repair did not restore the contact area or mean contact pressures to that of the intact knee or anatomic repair. However, an anatomic repair produced near-intact contact area and resulted in relatively minimal increases in mean and peak contact pressures compared with the intact knee. Papalia et al. [44] stated that biomechanical and clinical studies demonstrate that surgical repair of acute, traumatic meniscal root injuries fully restores the biomechanical features of the menisci, leading to pain relief and functional improvement.

3.3.1 Meniscectomy and Osteoarthritis

Fairbank [45] as early as 1948 reported radiographic changes in the knee after total meniscectomy, describing osteophyte formation, femoral condyle flattening and narrowing of joint space. Baratz et al. [46] demonstrated a decrease in tibiofemoral contact area by 10 % and an increase in peak local contact stress by 65 % with partial meniscectomy, and these values increased to 75 % and 235 %, respectively, in situations where total meniscectomy was done. Tapper and Hoover [47] stressed the importance of joint instability as a predisposing factor for joint osteoarthritis instability following total meniscectomy. Hsieh and Walker [48], Levy et al. [49] and Hollis et al. [50] also stressed the important function of the menisci as secondary stabilisers, particularly the medial meniscus in providing resistance to A-P translation in ACL-deficient knees.

3.4 Treatment

Treatment of meniscal tears has evolved from conservative to surgical, from open to arthroscopic technique and from total meniscectomy to partial meniscectomy and meniscal repair. Meniscal allograft transplant has also evolved as a salvage procedure to replicate the meniscal function.

3.4.1 Non-operative Treatment

Non-operative treatment is appropriate for minimally displaced degenerative tears and consists of activity modification, physical therapy, local ice packs and anti-inflammatory medication. Once the acute pain subsides, the patients are prescribed range-of-motion (ROM) exercises, and after attaining full ROM, any muscle imbalance is corrected [51]. If symptoms fail to settle, then arthroscopic surgery can be considered but is usually unnecessary.

3.4.2 Meniscectomy

Historically, the surgical treatment of an injured meniscus was open complete excision. Bland Suttons in 1897 had described the menisci as functionless remnants of intra-articular leg muscles. McMurray [52] advocated a total meniscectomy for any meniscal tear and had gone to the extent of stating that "a far too common error is shown in the incomplete removal of the injured meniscus". This philosophy was shown to be detrimental to the articular cartilage as described by Fairbanks in 1948, who described the changes in the knee joint following a meniscectomy which included ridge formation, narrowing of the joint space and flattening of the femoral condyle [53]. Further studies delineated the importance of preserving the meniscus as demonstrated by decreased contact areas and increased peak contact stress after a partial and/or total meniscectomy [54, 55]. Post meniscectomy, 74 % of knees had at least one Fairbank change and 39.4 % had degenerative arthritis as compared to 6 % of the contralateral normal knee [55]. Results of lateral meniscectomy are worse than that of medial meniscectomy, and resection of both menisci produced worse results than excision of a single meniscus. With the evolution of arthroscopic techniques, in the present day, almost all procedures related to the meniscus are done arthroscopically.

Meniscal tears in young patients and those associated with ACL tears should be repaired if at all possible. If the meniscus tear is complex and in an avascular zone, then it has no potential for healing, and a partial meniscectomy should be done. During a partial meniscectomy, unstable fragments should be removed to create a smooth transition, thus maintaining a functional meniscus. The short-term results of partial meniscectomy are excellent [56, 57]. Every attempt must be made to preserve as much of the meniscus as possible.

3.4.3 Meniscal Repair

The decision to repair a meniscus is dictated by the location of the tear [58, 59]. The indications for a meniscal repair are acute symptomatic tears: longitudinal orientation, peripheral red-on-red and red-on-white tears, greater than 10 mm in length with instability to probing and particularly with concomitant ACL reconstruction.

Chronic tears, degenerative tears, tears in the avascular zone and those associated with infection or rheumatoid arthritis have no potential for healing and are unsuitable for meniscal repair.

Meniscal repair includes inside-out techniques (Fig. 3.11), outside-in techniques and all-inside meniscal repair techniques.

The inside-out technique of meniscal repair is the gold standard and has given the best results to date. This technique is indicated for the tears of the body and posterior horn. A 73–91 % rate of success has been reported [60, 61]. Relook arthroscopies have demonstrated a 65–83 % rate of meniscal healing [62, 63]. Concomitant ACL reconstruction improves meniscal healing rates [64]. Meticulous adherence to surgical detail is a must to avoid neurological complications. Inside-out technique is suitable particularly for tears in the meniscal body, whereas the outside-in technique is required for anterior horn tears.

All-inside meniscal repair devices are increasingly being used because of shorter operating times, smaller incisions and the ability to be used in areas of the meniscus which

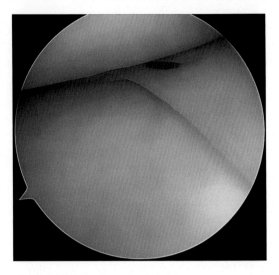

Fig. 3.11 Inside-out meniscal repair

are difficult to reach via an open procedure, particularly the posterior third of the meniscus. Many products have been available since the advent of this technique, and these include the Meniscus Arrow, T-Fix, S-D-sorb staple, Biostinger, Fastener, Clearfix screw, Dart, FAST-FIX, RapidLoc, MaxFire, Cinch and the Sequent. The newer devices are suture based and allow for compression across the meniscal tear. The success rate is around 85 % based on the published reports. As the follow-up increases, the failure rates increase too (0–43 %). Further studies are required to be able to formulate evidence-based guidelines for the use of all-inside devices for meniscal repair [65, 66].

Meniscal root tears are increasingly being identified as their significance in meniscal function is understood and recognised. Lateral meniscal root tears occur commonly with ACL tears. Medial meniscal root tears occur in a bimodal pattern. In the under-40 age group, they are seen in conjunction with other ligament tears secondary to sports injury, whereas in the over-40 age group, seemingly trivial trauma usually leads to these tears. Since the implication of a complete meniscal root lesion is complete loss of meniscal function, meniscal root repair is indicated in acute tears in younger patients to restore meniscal function [67, 68].

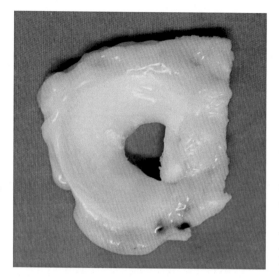

Fig. 3.12 Meniscal allograft

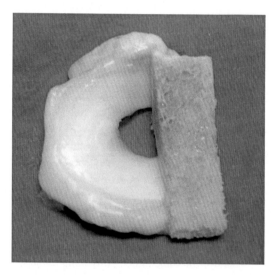

Fig. 3.13 Meniscal allograft with bone block

3.4.4 Meniscal Transplant (Figs. 3.12 and 3.13)

Patients who have had previous meniscectomy and have localised knee pain and functional disability secondary to meniscal deficiency may be appropriate for meniscal transplant.

Whilst meniscal repair is the treatment of choice whenever possible, this procedure is not possible for many complex meniscal tears and may result in complete loss of meniscal

function. This is particularly so for radial tears which extend to the meniscal rim. If the patient subsequently has recalcitrant localised pain in the meniscectomised compartment, meniscal allograft may be considered. The joint should be well aligned with minimal chondral wear to be appropriate for consideration.

Milachowski performed the first meniscal transplantation in 1984 in Munich University [69]; meniscal allografts have been found to be a feasible option for young patients with previously meniscectomised knees [70]. Menisci are 'immune privileged,' and studies have found little evidence of rejection [71]. The grafts readily heal at the repair site, and biomechanical testing has found that the grafts reduced joint forces compared to meniscectomy [72].

Four types of allografts are available:

Fresh
Fresh-frozen
Cryopreserved
Lyophilised (freeze-dried)

Viable donor cells in the transplanted meniscus are preserved only in fresh grafts and to a lesser extent in cryopreserved grafts. Deep freezing may denature histocompatibility antigens [73] and make a graft less immunogenic. Lyophilised grafts are prone to reduced tensile strength, graft shrinkage, poor rehydration and synovitis [74] and are best avoided.

Indications for allograft include young patients with prior meniscectomy with persistent pain in the involved compartment and with well-preserved articular cartilage, normal alignment and a stable joint [75]. Transplantation can also be considered in the presence of focal grade IV chondral changes, ligament instability or limb malalignment, provided these can be corrected prior to or during the surgery.

The use of allografts includes a potential for immune reactions and the risk of disease transmission. Although meniscus allografts are considered 'immune-privileged', they have been demonstrated to express class I and II histocompatibility antigens, which confer a potential for host immune response [76]. Bone plugs attached to the meniscal graft may increase the risk of immune reaction [77, 78].

Different methods for meniscus allotransplantation include both open and arthroscopic techniques, with or without the use of a bone block for lateral meniscus and bone plugs for medial meniscus. Arthroscopic techniques afford reduced surgical morbidity, avoid collateral ligament disruption and allow earlier rehabilitation. Biomechanical cadaver studies have shown superiority of a bony fixation over soft tissue fixation technique at the attachments of the meniscal horns [79–81]. However, with bone plugs/block, the implantation technique including allograft sizing is more exacting.

Correct size of the allograft is important for successful healing and functionality and to maximise the graft's potential capacity to be chondroprotective [82]. Knee joint tolerance for size mismatch is minimal, and graft size should be within 5 % of the original meniscus [83]. It is important to obtain an accurate attachment of the anterior and posterior horns of the transplant to the anatomically correct site of the tibial host and then secure attachment of the peripheral edge of the transplant to the host capsule. Exact cephalad or caudal attachment of the transplant to the host capsule is essential to prevent premature peripheral capsular separation and for recruitment of peripheral host soft tissue structures that will then restrain improper rotational and anterior translation.

Complications after this procedure are infrequent and include arthrofibrosis, loss of bony fixation, detachment of the allograft from the bone block, allograft tears and failure to heal.

3.5   Rehabilitation

Rehabilitation after meniscal surgery is tailored around the procedure performed. In case of a meniscal debridement or a partial meniscectomy, attention focuses on achieving full range of motion, strengthening of muscles and early return to full activity. Weight bearing as tolerated is started immediately after surgery. It is important to progress weight-bearing activities gradually to avoid development of overload symptoms, and

patients with significant meniscal deficiency should be counselled about the risk of arthritis and activity modifications that may be appropriate to reduce this risk.

In the event of a meniscal repair, restriction of weight bearing has not been shown to have any detrimental effect on meniscal healing, nor has progression of range of motion. For this reason, weight bearing and range of motion can usually be progressed as tolerated. Meniscal healing will most likely require a minimum of 3 months to approach normal strength, and it is sensible to avoid any forced passive flexion, running and twisting or pivoting activities during this period. A gradual return to sport can usually proceed after this period. When meniscal repair is done in conjunction with ACL reconstruction, the patient will usually follow a standard rehabilitation protocol. The only exception to these rules is meniscal root repairs which are under increased stress with weight bearing, which should therefore be restricted for approximately 6 weeks.

Conclusions

The menisci are critical to the function of the knee joint and have important roles in providing shock absorption, stability and joint lubrication. Meniscal tears can occur either as a result of acute injury or degeneration with age. Loss of meniscal tissue and associated function has significant implications, particularly in younger patients, and therefore, every attempt should be made to preserve meniscal tissue whenever possible either by avoiding unnecessary resection or performing meniscal repair. In the case of meniscal deficiency, patients should be counselled about the implications and advised carefully about management options to minimise the development of osteoarthritis particularly in the younger age groups.

References

1. Sutton JB. Ligaments: their nature and morphology. London: M. K. Lewis; 1987.
2. Mc Murray TP. The semi lunar cartilages. Br J Surg. 1942;29:407–14.

3. Gardner E, O'Rahilly R. The early development of the knee joint in staged human embryos. J Anat. 1968;102:289–99.
4. Mc Dermott LJ. Development of the human knee joint. Arch Surg. 1943;46:705.
5. Whillis J. The development of the synovial joint. J Anat (Lond). 1940;74:277–83.
6. Smillie IS. The congenital discoid meniscus. J Bone Joint Surg. 1948;30-B:671.
7. Nathan PA, Cole SC. Discoid meniscus. A clinical and pathologic study. Clin Orthop Relat Res. 1969;64:107–13.
8. Young RB. The external semilunar cartilage as a complete disc. In: Cleland J, Macke JY, Young RB, editors. Memoirs and memoranda in anatomy. London: Williams and Norgate; 1889.
9. Watanabe M, Takeda S, Ikeuchi H. Atlas of arthroscopy. Tokyo: Igaku-Shoin; 1978. p. 88.
10. Monllau JC, Leon A, Cugat R, Ballester J. The innervation of the human meniscus. Arthroscopy. 1998; 14:502–4.
11. Good CR, Green DW, Griffith MH, Valen AW, Widmann RF, Rodeo SA. Arthroscopic treatment of symptomatic discoid meniscus in children: classification, technique, and results. Arthroscopy. 2007;23:157–63.
12. Clark CR, Ogden JA. Development of the menisci of the human knee joint. J Bone Joint Surg Am. 1983; 65:538–47.
13. Herwig J, Egner E, Buddecke E. Chemical changes of human knee joint menisci in various stages of degeneration. Ann Rheum Dis. 1984;43:635–40.
14. Eyre DR, Wu JJ. Collagen of fibrocartilage: a distinctive molecular phenotype in bovine meniscus. FEBS Lett. 1983;158:265–70.
15. Bullough PG, Munuera L, Murphy J, et al. The strength of the menisci of the knee as it relates to their fine structure. J Bone Joint Surg. 1970;52B:564–7.
16. Fithian DC, Kelly MA, Mow VC. Material properties and structure function relationships in the menisci. Clin Orthop Relat Res. 1990;252:19–31.
17. Renstrom P, Johnson RJ. Anatomy and biomechanics of the menisci. Clin Sports Med. 1990;9:523.
18. Rath E, Richmond JC. The menisci: basic science and advances in treatment. Br J Sports Med. 2000; 34(4):252–7.
19. Arnoczky SP, Warren RF. Microvasculature of the human meniscus. Am J Sports Med. 1982;10(2):90–5.
20. King D. The function of the semilunar cartilages. J Bone Joint Surg. 1936;18-B:1069–76.
21. Fukubayashi T, Kurosawa H. The contact area and pressure distribution patter of the knee. A study of normal and osteoarthritic knee joints. Acta Orthop Scand. 1980;51:871–9.
22. Walker PS, Erkman MJ. The role of the menisci in force transmission across the knee. Clin Orthop Relat Res. 1975;109:184–92.
23. Johnson DL, Swenson TM, Livesay MS. Insertion site anatomy of the human menisci: gross, arthroscopic and topographical anatomy as a basis for meniscal transplantation. Arthroscopy. 1995;11:386.

24. Last RJ. Some anatomical details of the knee joint. J Bone Joint Surg Br. 1948;30:683.
25. Last RJ. The popliteus muscle and the lateral meniscus. J Bone Joint Surg Br. 1950;32:93.
26. Dickason JM, Del Pizzo W, Blazina ME. A series of 10 discoid medial menisci. Clin Orthop. 1992;168:75.
27. Schonholtz GJ, Koenig TM, Prince A. Bilateral discoid medial menisci: a case report and literature review. Arthroscopy. 1993;9:315.
28. Dickhaut SC, DeLee JC. The discoid lateral meniscus syndrome. J Bone Joint Surg Am. 1982;64:1068.
29. Ikeuchi H. Arthroscopic treatment of the discoid lateral meniscus: technique and long term results. Clin Orthop. 1983;176:225.
30. Washington III ER, Root L, Liener UC. Discoid lateral meniscus in children: long term follow up after excision. J Bone Joint Surg Am. 1995;77:1357.
31. Nielse AB, Yde J. Epidemiology of acute knee injuries: a prospective hospital investigation. J Trauma. 1991;31:1644–8.
32. Hede A, Jensen DB, Blyme P. Epidemiology of meniscal lesions in the knee: 1215 open operations in Copenhagen 1982–84. Acta Orthop Scand. 1990; 61:435–7.
33. Drosos GI, Pozo JL. The causes and mechanisms of meniscal injuries in the sporting and non sporting environment in an unselected population. Knee. 2004;11:143–9.
34. Poehling GG, Ruch DS, Chabon SJ. The landscape of meniscal injuries. Clin Sports Med. 1990;9:539–49.
35. Hegedus EJ, Cook C, Hasselblad V. Physical examination tests assessing a torn meniscus in the knee: a systematic review with meta-analysis. J Orthop Sports Phys Ther. 2007;37:541–50.
36. Meserve BB, Cleland JA, Boucher TR. A meta analysis examining clinical test utilities of assessing meniscal injury. Clin Rehabil. 2008;22:143–61.
37. Terry GC, Tagert BE, Young MJ. Reliability of the clinical assessment in predicting the cause of internal derangements of the knee. Arthroscopy. 1995;11:568–76.
38. Fu F. Master techniques in orthopaedic surgery; sports medicine. 3rd ed. Lippincott William Wilkins; Philadelphia, USA. 2010.
39. Cooper DE, Arnoczky SP, Warren RF. Meniscal repair. Clin Sports Med. 1991;10(3):529–48.
40. Anderson AF, et al. Interobserver Reliability of the International Society of Arthroscopy, Knee Surgery and Orthopaedic Sports Medicine (ISAKOS) Classification of Meniscal Tears. Am J Sports Med. 2011;39(5):926–32.
41. Guermazi A, et al. Medial posterior meniscal root tears are associated with development or worsening of medial tibiofemoral cartilage damage: the multicenter osteoarthritis study. Radiology. 2013;268(3):814–21.
42. LaPrade CM, James EW, Cram TR, et al. Meniscal root tears: a classification system based on tear morphology. Am J Sports Med. 2015;43(2):363–9.
43. LaPrade CM, Foad A, Smith SD, et al. Biomechanical consequences of a nonanatomic posterior medial meniscal root repair. Am J Sports Med. 2015;43(4):912–20.

44. Papalia R, Vasta S, Franceschi F, et al. Meniscal root tears: from basic science to ultimate surgery. Br Med Bull. 2013;106:91–115.
45. Fairbank TJ. Knee joint changes after meniscectomy. J Bone Joint Surg Br. 1948;30:664–70.
46. Baratz ME, Fu F, Mengato R. Meniscal tears: the effect of meniscectomy and of repair on intraarticulaar contact areas and stress in the human knee: a preliminary report. Am J Sports Med. 1986;14:270–5.
47. Tapper EM, Hoover NW. Late results after meniscectomy. J Bone Joint Surg Am. 1969;51:517–26.
48. Hsieh HH, Walker PS. Stabilizing mechanisms of the loaded and unloaded knee joint. J Bone Joint Surg Am. 1976;58:87–93.
49. Levy MI, Torzilli PA, Warren RF. The effect of medial meniscectomy on anterior-posterior motion of the knee. J Bone Joint Surg Am. 1982;64:883–8.
50. Hollis JM, Pearsall AW, Niciforos PG. Change in meniscal strain with anterior cruciate ligament injury and after reconstruction. Am J Sports Med. 2000;28:700–4.
51. Insall JN, Scott WN. Surgery of the knee. 4th ed. Churchill Livingstone. Elsevier, Philadelphia, USA. 2006.
52. McMurray TP. The semilunar cartilages. Br J Surg. 1942;29:407–14.
53. Fairbanks TJ. Knee joint changes after meniscectomy. J Bone Joint Surg Br. 1948;30:664–70.
54. Kruger-Franke M, Siebert CH, Kugler A, et al. Late results after arthroscopic partial medial meniscectomy. Knee Surg Sports Traumatol Arthrosc. 1999;7:81–4.
55. Johnson RJ, Kettelkamp DB, Clark W, Leaverton P. Factors affecting late results after meniscectomy. J Bone Joint Surg Am. 1974;56:719–29.
56. Jareguito JW, Elliot JS, Leitner T, et al. The effects of partial lateral meniscectomy in an otherwise normal knee: a retrospective review of functional, clinical and radiographic results. Arthroscopy. 1995;11:29–36.
57. Burks RT, Metcalf MH, Metcalf RW. Fifteen year follow up of arthroscopic partial meniscectomy. Arthroscopy. 1997;13:673–9.
58. Dehaven KE. Decision making factors in the treatment of meniscus lesions. Clin Orthop. 1990;252:49–54.
59. Newman AP, Daniels AU, Burks RT. Principles and decision making in meniscal surgery. Arthroscopy. 1993;9:33–51.
60. Barber FA. Meniscus repair: results of an arthroscopic technique. Arthroscopy. 1987;3:25–30.
61. Jorgensen U, Sonne-Holm S, Lauridsen F, et al. Long term follow up of meniscectomy in atheletes. A prospective longitudinal study. J Bone Joint Surg Br. 1987;69(1):80–3.
62. Horibe S, Shino K, Nakata K, et al. Second look arthroscopy after meniscal repair: a review of 132 menisci repaired by an arthroscopic inside out technique. J Bone Joint Surg Br. 1995;77:245–9.
63. Rubman MH, Noyes FR, Barber-Westin SD. Arthroscopic repair of meniscal tears that extend into the avascular zone. A review of 198 single and complex tears. Am J Sports Med. 1999;26:87–95.
64. Ranalletta M, Rossi W, Paterno M, et al. An arthroscopic study in anterior cruciate ligament deficient knees. Arthroscopy. 2007;23(3):275–7.
65. Gill SS, Diduch DR. Outcomes after meniscal repair using the meniscus arrow in knees undergoing concurrent anterior cruciate ligament reconstruction. Arthroscopy. 2002;18:569–77.
66. Lozano J, Ma C, Cannon W. All inside meniscal repair: a systematic review. Clin Orthop Relat Res. 2006;455:134–41.
67. Beasley L, Armfield RD, West RV, et al. Medial meniscus root tears: an unsolved problem- demographic, radiographic and arthroscopic findings. Pittsburgh Orthop J. 2005;16:155.
68. Habata T, Uematsu K, Hattori K, et al. Clinical features of the posterior horn tear in the medial meniscus. Arch Orthop Trauma Surg. 2004;124:642–5.
69. Milachowski KA, Weismeier K, Wirth CJ. Homologous meniscal transplantation. Experimental and clinical results. Int Orthop. 1989;13:1–9.
70. Aglietti P, Buzzi R, Bassi PB. Arthroscopic partial meniscectomy in the anterior cruciate ligament deficient patient. Am J Sports Med. 1988;16:597–602.
71. Rijk PC. Meniscal allograft transplantation – part I : background, results, graft selection and preservation, and surgical considerations. Arthroscopy. 2004;20:728–43.
72. Siegel MG, Robert CS. Meniscal allografts. Clin Sports Med. 1993;12:59–80.
73. Brown KL, Cruess RL. Bone and cartilage transplantation in orthopaedic surgery. A review. J Bone Joint Surg Am. 1982;64:270–9.
74. Jackson DW, Windler GE, Simon TM. Intraarticular reaction associated with the use of freeze-dried, ethylene oxide-sterilized bone-patella tendon-bone allografts in the reconstruction of the anterior cruciate ligament. Am J Sports Med. 1990;18:1–11.
75. Hamlet W, Liu SH, Yang R. Destruction of a cryopreserved meniscal allograft: a case for acute rejection. Arthroscopy. 1997;13:517–21.
76. Khoury MA, Goldberg VM, Stevenson S. Demonstration of HLA and ABH antigens in fresh and frozen human menisci by immunohistochemistry. J Orthop Res. 1994;12:751–7.
77. Bos GD, Goldberg VM, Zika JM, Heiple KG, Powell AE. Immune responses of rats to frozen bone allografts. J Bone Joint Surg Am. 1983;65:239–46.
78. Stevenson S. The immune response to osteochondral allografts in dogs. J Bone Joint Surg Am. 1987;69:573–82.
79. Chen MI, Branch TP, Hutton WC. Is it important to secure the horns during lateral meniscal transplantation? A cadaveric study. Arthroscopy. 1996;12:174–81.
80. Paletta Jr GA, Manning T, Snell E, Parker R, Bergfeld J. The effect of allograft meniscal replacement on intraarticular contact area and pressures in the human knee: a biomechanical study. Am J Sports Med. 1997;25:692–8.
81. Alhalki MM, Howell SM, Hull ML. How three methods for fixing a medial meniscal autograft affect tibial contact mechanics. Am J Sports Med. 1999;27:320–8.
82. Verdonk R, Kohn D. Harvest and conservation of meniscal allografts. Scand J Med Sci Sports. 1999;9:158–9.
83. Wilcox TR, Goble EM, Doucette SA. Goble technique of meniscus transplantation. Am J Knee Surg. 1996;9:37–42.

Arthroscopic Debridement of the Knee in the Presence of Osteoarthritis

Myles R.J. Coolican and Kunal Dhurve

Contents

M.R.J. Coolican, MD, FRACS (✉)
K. Dhurve, MS (Ortho)
Sydney Orthopaedic Research Institute,
Chatswood, NSW, Australia
e-mail: mcoolican@sydneyortho.com.au

This chapter presents evidence to help answer the question as to whom, if anyone, with knee arthritis should undergo knee arthroscopy and provides recommendations on alternative treatments.

4.1 The History of Joint Debridement

Debridement of the knee joint for osteoarthritis was first described in English literature by Haggart in 1940 [1, 2] and by Magnuson in 1941 [3].

Pridie [4] presented to the British Orthopaedic Association in 1959 the results of his findings with re-exploration of four knees after previous extensive debridement that included drilling with a 0.25 in. drill bit into sclerotic bare bone on the medial condyle. The findings in the four patients whose surgery had not successfully relieved symptoms showed that the previously bare medial femoral condyle was covered by fibrocartilage. Insall reported the results of Dr Pridie's work in 1967 [5]. The patients had an average age of 53 years, and after the surgery, 79 % functioned with little or no pain and 84 % flexed to 90° or more. Seventy-seven per cent of the patients thought the operation was a success. Pridie, as well as Haggart and Magnuson, emphasised the importance of correct patient selection in performing knee debridement. The patients were more likely to be happy with their operation if they were middle aged, robust, and capable of a vigorous rehabilitation programme.

D.A. Parker (ed.), *Management of Knee Osteoarthritis in the Younger, Active Patient: An Evidence-Based Practical Guide for Clinicians*, DOI 10.1007/978-3-662-48530-9_4

There were subsequently few other reports of the results of open debridement, and it is an operation that did not stand the test of time. The advent of joint arthroplasty in the 1970s replaced joint debridement, and around this time, arthroscopic surgery that had developed in Japan in the first half of the twentieth century gradually became more popular and widespread in Europe, North and South America, and Australasia. Until the 1960s, it was a surgical procedure confined largely to Japan. Not surprisingly, the advent of arthroscopy saw a resurgence of joint debridement for osteoarthritis particularly in patients whose symptoms and radiographic wear were not considered sufficiently advanced to merit joint replacement. The enthusiasm for arthroscopic treatment of the mild to moderately arthritic knee in the 1980s and 1990s was unprecedented given its lower morbidity compared with open debridement. But, it should also be pointed out that an operation that by and large had at the most moderate success as an open procedure would likely have much the same results when performed with the lower morbidity arthroscopic procedure. Subsequent years have seen the publication of several well-conducted trials evaluating the efficacy of arthroscopic knee surgery for osteoarthritis and have shown arthroscopic debridement to be no better than other non-operative treatments. Whilst the results of these studies are well recognised in the orthopaedic community, there has been surprisingly little alteration in the rates of surgery across the globe.

4.2   Trends in the Rate of Arthroscopic Knee Surgery

Wai et al. [6] published in 2002 a study of the incidence of arthroscopy from 1992 to 1996 in Canada (Fig. 4.1). It was a population-based comparison of patients over the age of 50 undergoing arthroscopic surgery. At 12 months following arthroscopic surgery, 9.2 % of patients had undergone a total knee replacement, and this figure was 19 % for those over the age of 70.

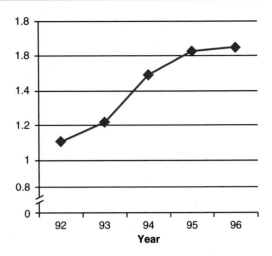

Fig. 4.1 Age and gender-adjusted population rates (per 1000) of arthroscopic knee debridement by year [6]

Hawker et al. [7] in 2008 published a population-based comparison of the incidence of arthroscopy in Bristol, UK, and Ontario, Canada, for the years 1993, 1997, 2002, and 2004. Whilst the performance of arthroscopy mostly increased over time in both nations, there was a fall in Ontario between 1993 and 1997 followed by an increase. The authors compared the incidence of arthroscopy in each of the four income quartiles for both regions and found that the highest rate of arthroscopy was in the higher income quartile for both nations. In Bristol, 4.8 % of the patients progressed to a total knee replacement over the subsequent 12 months, and for Ontario, Canada, this figure was 8.5 %. In the same years in Bristol, 2.7 % of all patients undergoing total knee replacement had undergone an arthroscopic procedure in the prior 12 months, and in Canada this figure was 5.7 %.

Dearing and Brenkel [8] in 2010 looked at the incidence of arthroscopy across 15 health regions in Scotland. They described a marked regional variation from a high of 36 arthroscopies per 100,000 population to a low of 5. The authors also reported on the incidence of total knee replacement in the same period within each region and demonstrated a poor match on the incidence of arthroscopy and total knee replacement. This work did not indicate if the incidence of arthroscopy was related to patient-surgeon ratios.

Harris et al. [9] reported in 2013 on the incidence of arthroscopy in Australia. Whilst there have been a steady number of total arthroscopies performed in the period 2000–2008, there has been a slight decline in the public sector and an increase in the private sector. Interestingly, these rates are approximately ten times the greatest incidence of arthroscopy performed in Tasmania. The age groups from 45 to 64 and 65 to 74 show an increasing rate, whilst other age groups are declining. The conversion rate to a total knee replacement within 24 months of total knee replacement declined from 23.2 % in 2000 to 20.1 % in 2006.

Bohensky et al. [10] utilised rates of total knee replacement for comparison with the incidence of arthroscopy rather than relying on population base alone, their reasoning being that rates of all types of knee surgery are increasing and the rate of TKR could be an indexed comparison. Whilst this group demonstrated a decrease in arthroscopy rates overall in the period 2000–2009, there was no decrease in patients with a diagnosis of arthritis undergoing arthroscopic surgery.

A summary of the trends in arthroscopic knee surgery would indicate that across the globe, orthopaedic surgeons are performing arthroscopic knee surgery at the same or greater rates in the past 15 years with a marked regional variation not necessarily explained by surgeon numbers or method of remuneration. Over 20 % of patients aged greater than 60 years undergoing knee arthroscopy have a total knee performed within 2 years, and it is likely that the arthroscopic surgery was either unnecessary or possibly contributed to the deterioration of the knee.

4.3 Literature Review Arthroscopic Lavage

The principle of arthroscopic lavage is to remove chondral debris, loose synovial fragments, and synovial fluid with associated inflammatory cytokines from the joint. This can be achieved with either separate inflow or outflow points through two portals, or lavage may be tidal with variations in volume of fluid and length of time it is in contact with the joint.

Earlier observational studies suggested there were benefits to knee lavage. Livesley et al. [11] in 1991 showed significant benefit of washout over physiotherapy, and Jackson and Dieterichs [12] in 2003 reported a retrospective series of significant relief lasting 1–5 years after washout.

In 2000, Kalunian et al. [13] published a multicentre randomised double-blind placebo controlled trial of 90 patients. Group 1 received arthroscopic irrigation with 3000 ml, whilst group 2, the placebo group, received 250 ml of arthroscopic irrigation. There was improvement in pain at 12 months in favour of full irrigation which was found to be of particular benefit in patients with crystal arthropathy.

A Cochrane review published by Reichenbach et al. [14] in 2010 included seven small series. There was little evidence in these series of benefit in pain relief or function at 3 months and at 1 year with the authors commenting that trials with a sham procedure that closely mimicked lavage showed a clear null effect. The small improvements seen in some trials at 1 year may be due to chance. Arthroscopic lavage for the treatment of osteoarthritis was not recommended.

4.4 Arthroscopic Debridement for Osteoarthritis

Arthroscopic debridement of the knee has been practised since arthroscopy became a popular procedure in the 1970s. Success rate for arthroscopic debridement of the osteoarthritic knee range from 40 to 75 % with multiple authors – Baumgaertner et al. [15], 1990; Harwin [16], 1999; Hubbard [17], 1996; McGinley et al. [18], 1999; McLaren et al. [19], 1991; Shannon et al. [20], 2001; Sprague [21], 1981; and Timoney et al. [22], 1990, all reporting good outcomes with pain relief and function. Some of these authors (Baumgaertner, Shannon, Timoney, Hubbard, and McLaren) showed that palliative effects were maintained for 2–5 years with McGinley, Harwin, and Aicroth, 1999; Fond et al. [23], 2002; and Dervin et al. [24], 2003, showing the palliative effects were maintained for between 7 and 13 years. Predictors of a positive outcome were young patients with a short duration of symptoms who had early osteo-arthritis on radiographs without malalignment and who had mechanical symptoms.

Two randomised trials were published in the 1990s comparing arthroscopic debridement to lavage. Chang et al. [25] in 1993 reported on 18 patients who underwent arthroscopic debridement compared with 14 patients who underwent joint lavage using a tidal system. This was to our knowl-edge the first published study to cast doubt on the efficacy of arthroscopic debridement to treat osteoarthritis. A single-blinded assessor was uti-lised at each site with outcome assessments being made at 3 and 12 months utilising the pain and functional status scales from the Arthritis Impact Measurement System (AIMS). Withdrawals at the 12-month mark were 22 % for the arthroscopy group and 7 % of the lavage group. There were no statistically significant differences between the groups at 3 months and 12 months.

Hubbard [17] compared 14 patients undergoing arthroscopic debridement with 36 undergoing a washout for 'degeneration of the medial femoral condyle'. Pain and function were measured with the Lysholm score. The outcome assessors were neither independent nor blinded with the loss to follow-up being 20 % of the debridement group and 28 % for the washout group. There was a sig-nificant difference in pain relief at 1 and 5 years in favour of the arthroscopic debridement group.

In 2002, Moseley et al. [26] published a blinded control trial in which there were three groups, 59 patients underwent arthroscopic debridement, 61 underwent arthroscopic lavage, and 60 had placebo surgery with a short-acting IV tranquiliser and an opioid. In the placebo group where the patients were partially con-scious, they were kept in the operating theatre for the same amount of time as arthroscopic debride-ment, and flushing sounds and requests for instru-ments by the surgeon were made to mimic arthroscopic lavage or surgery. Of the 324 eligi-ble patients (mostly male veterans), 56 % partici-pated possibly producing a selection bias. There was a 10 % loss to follow-up in each group with results being presented on 163 patients who com-pleted the trial to 2 years follow-up. Pain was measured with the Knee Society pain score,

physical function with the AIMS 2, and SF36 at week 2 and week 6 and at the 3, 6, 12, and 24 months mark. There was no statistically signifi-cant difference between the arthroscopic debride-ment and the lavage group. There were however differences between the arthroscopic group and the placebo with these reaching significance favouring the placebo group at the 2 weeks and 12 months. Other than at the 18-month mark, the placebo group scored higher on the mean knee-specific pain scale score and the AIMS 2 walking-bending subscale across the 2-year period. Criticisms of this study included that non-vali-dated measurement scales were utilised, and in addition, there was no non-operative comparative group.

In 2008, Kirkley et al. [27] published a single-centre randomised control trial comparing two groups. The treatment group underwent a combi-nation of knee lavage and arthroscopic debride-ment followed by optimised medical and physical therapy for osteoarthritis of the knee. The control group had optimised medical and physical ther-apy alone. Of the 188 patients who randomised, 168 completed the study with a participation rate of 89 %. There were a number of exclusion crite-ria including patients with bucket-handle menis-cal tears, Kellgren-Lawrence grade 4 in 2 compartments, prior arthroscopy for knee arthri-tis, and varus deformity greater than 5°. WOMAC and SF36 were utilised to measure outcomes. The groups were similar in their use of medical therapy including non-steroidals, paracetamol, chondroitin, and hyaluronic acid injections as well as participation in physiotherapy. Although the arthroscopic group started with a worse (higher) mean WOMAC score, there were no sig-nificant differences between the two groups at all time points. A separate analysis between surgical and non-surgical management was made for sev-eral subgroups. Patients with Kellgren-Lawrence grade 2 (milder wear) had no better results with surgery than the non-operative group, and simi-larly, there was no benefit with surgery in Kellgren-Lawrence grades 3 and 4 (more advanced wear) or in patients with mechanical symptoms such as catching and locking. The authors' conclusion was that arthroscopic surgery for osteoarthritis of the knee provided no additional benefit to optimised physical and medical therapy.

A Cochrane review by Laupattarakasem et al. [28] in 2008 concluded that there is 'gold' level evidence that arthroscopic debridement has no benefit for undiscriminated osteoarthritis whether the symptoms are a consequence of a mechanical or an inflammatory cause.

4.5   Arthroscopic Meniscectomy for Degenerative Tears with Little or No Osteoarthritis

Whilst it is accepted by most orthopaedic surgeons that arthroscopy has an extremely limited role in the management of osteoarthritis, arthroscopic surgery for degenerative tears of the meniscus in the presence of little or no osteoarthritis is a commonly performed procedure. There is some doubt as to whether this procedure is always necessary with studies demonstrating physical therapy may resolve symptoms in a majority of patients. In 2013, Sihvonen et al. [29] published a multicentre randomised double-blind sham-controlled trial of 146 patients without osteoarthritis who were suffering degenerative medial meniscal tears. The patients were randomised to arthroscopy or sham surgery. Patients were followed up at 2, 6, and 12 months. The Lysholm score was identical for the patients at baseline and at the 2, 6, and 12 months, whilst the WOMET score was very similar at baseline and higher (favourable) for the arthroscopic meniscectomy group at 2 and 6 months, but at 12 months the groups were the same. A similar pattern was seen with pain after exercise in the two groups being similar at baseline, better at 2 and 6 months in the arthroscopic partial meniscectomy group and identical at 12 months. The conclusion after this trial involving patients without knee osteoarthritis but with symptoms of a degenerative medial meniscal tear was that the outcomes after arthroscopic partial meniscectomy are no better than those after a sham surgical procedure.

Herrlin et al. [30] reported in 2007 and again in 2013 [31] on a prospective randomised study of patients with a degenerative medial meniscal tear without osteoarthritis. A feature of these studies is patients declining to participate with the non-participation rate being 41 %. Non-traumatic meniscal tears were divided into two groups: those that underwent arthroscopic partial medial meniscectomy followed by physiotherapy/exercise and those who underwent physiotherapy/exercise alone. KOOS, Tegner, Lysholm, and a visual analog scale were utilised to measure outcomes. Whilst the arthroscopy and exercise group scored slightly better on all KOOS scales than exercise alone, both were substantially improved. At 8 weeks the scores were similar for both the arthroscopic/exercise group and the exercise alone group and this continued at 6 months. The authors' conclusion was that there was no significant benefit from meniscectomy using any of the outcome measures at 8 weeks and 6 months. A further publication from Herrlin et al. [31] on the same group of patients reported the results of the same cohort at 2 and 5 years after the intervention. This showed that both groups enjoyed highly significant clinical improvements from baseline to follow-ups at 2 and 5 years on all subscales of KOOS as well as the Lysholm score and VAS. However, there were no differences between the groups. It is important to point out that one third of the patients who were treated with exercise therapy alone were unimproved after this treatment but were improved after arthroscopic surgery. The authors conclude that exercise therapy can be recommended as an initial treatment with arthroscopy reserved for those who failed to improve and that this group of patients who undergo delayed surgery achieve the same results as those who were immediately randomised to surgery.

4.6   Evidence-Based Guidelines and Statements

A review of past and current evidence-based guidelines for the treatment of osteoarthritis with surgery – either lavage or debridement – shows a gradual alteration from reluctance to recommend lavage to specific recommendations against this surgery.

In 2008, guidelines issued by the British National Health Service, National Institute for Health and Clinical Excellence (NICE) [32], concluded that evidence on the safety and efficacy of arthroscopic knee washout with debridement for the treatment of osteoarthritis is adequate to support the use of this procedure provided that normal arrangements are in place for consent, audit, and clinical governance. The 2008 guidelines also suggested that current evidence showed that arthroscopic knee washout alone should not be used as a treatment for osteoarthritis because it could not demonstrate a benefit in the short or long term. In 2014, an update on these guidelines was more specific stating that patients should not be referred for arthroscopic lavage or debridement as part of treatment for osteoarthritis unless the patient with knee arthritis has a clear history of mechanical locking, as opposed to morning stiffness, giving way or X-ray evidence of loose bodies [33].

Guidelines issued jointly by the British Orthopaedic Association, the British Association for Surgery of the Knee, the Combined Charter of Physiotherapy, and the Royal College of Surgeons of England in 2013 stated that knee arthroscopy, lavage, and debridement should be considered in patients with a clear history of mechanical symptoms, for example, locking, who have not responded to at least 3 months of non-surgical treatment. This group also recommended arthroscopy when a detailed understanding of the degree of compartment damage within the knee is required above that demonstrated by imaging, for example, when considering patients for surgical intervention such as a high tibial osteotomy. The guidelines also concluded that knee arthroscopy, lavage, and debridement should not be offered to patients with the non-mechanical symptoms of pain and stiffness.

The Australian Knee Society, after a review of the literature and consensus meeting in 2014, published on its website a series of statements concerning arthroscopic treatment for osteoarthritis of the knee as presented below.

Arthroscopic debridement and/or lavage have been shown to have no beneficial effect on the natural history of osteoarthritis. Nor is it indicated as a primary treatment in the management of osteoar-

thritis. Notwithstanding, this does not preclude the use of arthroscopic surgery where indicated to manage symptomatic coexisting pathology in the presence of osteoarthritis.

There are certain clinical scenarios in which arthroscopic surgery, in the presence of osteoarthritis, may be appropriate – albeit after considered discussion with the patient. These include, but are not necessarily limited to, the following:

- Known or suspected septic arthritis
- Unstable meniscal tears after an appropriate trial of non-operative treatment
- Symptomatic loose bodies
- Meniscal tears that require repair
- Inflammatory arthropathy requiring synovectomy
- Synovial pathology requiring biopsy or resection
- Unstable chondral pathology causing mechanical symptoms
- As an adjunct to, and in combination with, other surgical procedures as appropriate for osteoarthritis: for example, high tibial osteotomy and patello femoral realignment
- Diagnostic arthroscopy when the diagnosis is unclear on MRI

The American Academy of Orthopaedic Surgeons 2nd Edition Evidence-Based Guidelines for Treatment of Osteoarthritis of the Knee rates the strength of their advice based on available knowledge as either strong or inconclusive [34]. Their Recommendation 12 in May 2013 states 'we cannot recommend performing arthroscopy with lavage and/or debridement in patients with a primary diagnosis of symptomatic osteoarthritis of the knee. Strength of recommendation: strong'. In Recommendation 13, 'we are able to recommend for or against arthroscopic partial meniscectomy in patients with osteoarthritis of the knee with a torn meniscus. Strength of recommendation: inconclusive'.

4.7 Summary and Conclusions

The role of arthroscopic surgery to manage osteoarthritis of the knee is extremely limited and has been shown to be no more effective than sham surgery. However, its use as a treatment modality continues across the globe. A summary of current evidence-based guidelines from multiple respected national bodies recommends against the use of arthroscopy as a treatment for knee osteoarthritis. Patients with a degenerative medial meniscal tear should undergo surgery if the symptoms are not relieved by a structured physiotherapy programme including resistance exercises, and approximately one third of these patients will require surgery.

References

1. Haggart GE. The surgical treatment of degenerative arthritis of the knee joint. J Bone Joint Surg. 1940;22(3):717–29.
2. Haggart GE. Surgical treatment of degenerative arthritis of the knee joint. N Engl J Med. 1947;236(26):971–3.
3. Magnuson PB. Joint debridement. Surgical treatment of degenerative arthritis. J Surg Gynecol Obstet. 1941;73:1–9.
4. Pridie K. A method of resurfacing knee joints: proceedings of the British Orthopaedic Association. J Bone Joint Surg Br. 1959;41:618.
5. Insall JN. Intra-articular surgery for degenerative arthritis of the knee. A report of the work of the late K. H. Pridie. J Bone Joint Surg Br. 1967;49(2):211–28.
6. Wai EK, Kreder HJ, Williams JI. Arthroscopic debridement of the knee for osteoarthritis in patients fifty years of age or older: utilization and outcomes in the Province of Ontario. J Bone Joint Surg Am. 2002;84-A(1):17–22.
7. Hawker G, Guan J, Judge A, Dieppe P. Knee arthroscopy in England and Ontario: patterns of use, changes over time, and relationship to total knee replacement. J Bone Joint Surg Am. 2008;90(11):2337–45.
8. Dearing J, Brenkel IJ. Incidence of knee arthroscopy in patients over 60 years of age in Scotland. Surgeon. 2010;8(3):144–50.
9. Harris IA, Madan NS, Naylor JM, Chong S, Mittal R, Jalaludin BB. Trends in knee arthroscopy and subsequent arthroplasty in an Australian population: a retrospective cohort study. BMC Musculoskelet Disord. 2013;14(1):143.
10. Bohensky MA, Sundararajan V, Andrianopoulos N, de Steiger RN, Bucknill A, Kondogiannis CM, McColl G, Brand CA. Trends in elective knee arthroscopies in a population-based cohort, 2000–2009. Med J Aust. 2012;197(7):399–403.
11. Livesley P, Doherty M, Needoff M, Moulton A. Arthroscopic lavage of osteoarthritic knees. J Bone Joint Surg Br Vol. 1991;73-B(6):922–6.
12. Jackson RW, Dieterichs C. The results of arthroscopic lavage and debridement of osteoarthritic knees based on the severity of degeneration. Arthroscopy. 2003; 19(1):13–20.
13. Kalunian K, Moreland L, Klashman D, Brion P, Concoff A, Myers S, Singh R, Ike R, Seeger L, Rich E. Visually-guided irrigation in patients with early knee osteoarthritis: a multicenter randomized, controlled trial. Osteoarthritis Cartilage. 2000;8(6):412–8.
14. Reichenbach S, Rutjes AW, Nüesch E, Trelle S, Jüni P. Joint lavage for osteoarthritis of the knee. Cochrane Database Syst Rev. 2010;12(5):1–45.
15. Baumgaertner MR, Cannon WD, Vittori JM, Schmidt ES, Maurer RC. Arthroscopic debridement of the arthritic knee. Clin Orthop Relat Res. 1990;253: 197–202.
16. Harwin SF. Arthroscopic debridement for osteoarthritis of the knee: predictors of patient satisfaction. Arthroscopy. 1999;15(2):142–6.
17. Hubbard M. Articular debridement versus washout for degeneration of the medial femoral condyle. A five-year study. J Bone Joint Surg Br Vol. 1996; 78(2):217–9.
18. McGinley BJ, Cushner FD, Scott WN. Debridement arthroscopy 10-year followup. Clin Orthop Relat Res. 1999;367:190–4.
19. McLaren A, Blokker C, Fowler P, Roth J, Rock M. Arthroscopic debridement of the knee for osteoarthrosis. Canadian J Surg J Canadien de chirurgie. 1991;34(6):595–8.
20. Shannon F, Devitt A, Poynton A, Fitzpatrick P, Walsh M. Short-term benefit of arthroscopic washout in degenerative arthritis of the knee. Int Orthop. 2001;25(4):242–5.
21. Sprague NF. Arthroscopic debridement for degenerative knee joint disease. Clin Orthop Relat Res. 1981;160:118–23.
22. Timoney J, Kneisl J, Barrack R, Alexander A. Arthroscopy update# 6. Arthroscopy in the osteoarthritic knee. Long-term follow-up. Orthop Rev. 1990;19(4):371–3. 376–379.
23. Fond J, Rodin D, Ahmad S, Nirschl RP. Arthroscopic debridement for the treatment of osteoarthritis of the knee: 2-and 5-year results. Arthroscopy. 2002; 18(8):829–34.
24. Dervin GF, Stiell IG, Rody K, Grabowski J. Effect of arthroscopic débridement for osteoarthritis of the knee on health-related quality of life*. J Bone Joint Surg. 2003;85(1):10–9.
25. Chang RW, Falconer J, David Stulberg S, Arnold WJ, Manheim LM, Dyer AR. A randomized, controlled trial of arthroscopic surgery versus closed-needle joint lavage for patients with osteoarthritis of the knee. Arthritis Rheum. 1993;36(3):289–96.
26. Moseley JB, O'Malley K, Petersen NJ, Menke TJ, Brody BA, Kuykendall DH, Hollingsworth JC, Ashton CM, Wray NP. A controlled trial of arthroscopic surgery for osteoarthritis of the knee. N Engl J Med. 2002;347(2):81–8.
27. Kirkley A, Birmingham TB, Litchfield RB, Giffin JR, Willits KR, Wong CJ, Feagan BG, Donner A, Griffin SH, D'Ascanio LM. A randomized trial of arthroscopic surgery for osteoarthritis of the knee. N Engl J Med. 2008;359(11):1097–107.
28. Laupattarakasem W, Laopaiboon M, Laupattarakasem P, Sumananont C. Arthroscopic debridement for knee osteoarthritis. Cochrane Database Syst Rev. 2008; 23(1):1–32.
29. Sihvonen R, Paavola M, Malmivaara A, Itälä A, Joukainen A, Nurmi H, Kalske J, Järvinen

TL. Arthroscopic partial meniscectomy versus sham surgery for a degenerative meniscal tear. N Engl J Med. 2013;369(26):2515–24.

30. Herrlin S, Hallander M, Wange P, Weidenhielm L, Werner S. Arthroscopic or conservative treatment of degenerative medial meniscal tears: a prospective randomised trial. Knee Surg Sports Traumatol Arthrosc. 2007;15(4):393–401.

31. Herrlin SV, Wange PO, Lapidus G, Hallander M, Werner S, Weidenhielm L. Is arthroscopic surgery beneficial in treating non-traumatic, degenerative

medial meniscal tears? A five year follow-up. Knee Surg Sports Traumatol Arthrosc. 2013;21(2):358–64.

32. Conaghan PG, Dickson J, Grant RL. Guidelines: care and management of osteoarthritis in adults: summary of NICE guidance. BMJ. 2008;336(7642):502.

33. NICE National Institute for Health and Care Excellence osteoarthritis: care and management in adults. NICE clinical guideline 117. February 2014.

34. Jevsevar DS. Treatment of osteoarthritis of the knee: evidence-based guideline. J Am Acad Orthop Surg. 2013;21(9):571–6.

Cartilage Preservation and Restoration Techniques: Evidence-Based Practice

Brian M. Devitt, Stuart W. Bell,
and Tim S. Whitehead

Contents

B.M. Devitt
Director of Research OrthoSport Victoria Research Unit, OrthoSport Victoria, Level 5, 89 Bridge Road, Epworth Richmond, VIC 3121, Australia

S.W. Bell
Consultant Orthopaedic Surgeon, Royal Alexandra Hospital, Corsebar Road, Paisley, PA29PN, United Kingdom

T.S. Whitehead (✉)
OrthoSport Victoria,
Level 5, 89 Bridge Road, Richmond,
VIC 3121, Australia
e-mail: TSWhitehead@osv.com.au

5.1 Introduction

The optimum treatment of a full-thickness defect of knee articular cartilage in a young symptomatic patient remains controversial and represents a significant challenge for orthopaedic surgeons. Full-thickness articular cartilage defects have limited intrinsic capacity for repair [1]. Moreover, it has been shown that patients with isolated symptomatic cartilage defects awaiting treatment have similar quality-of-life scores as patients with knee osteoarthritis awaiting total knee arthroplasty or knee osteotomies and worse clinical scores than patients awaiting anterior cruciate ligament (ACL) reconstruction [2]. For symptomatic defects refractory to conservative management, operative intervention can provide both pain relief and functional improvement [3, 4].

5.1.1 Cartilage and Osteoarthritis

The health of articular cartilage and the development of osteoarthritis are integrally linked. Osteoarthritis is a degenerative joint disease characterised primarily by progressive breakdown of articular cartilage [5]. A strong correlation exists between increasing age and the prevalence of osteoarthritis, which is one of the most common causes of pain and disability in middle-aged and older people [6]. Evidence focusing on age-related changes in the function of chondrocytes

D.A. Parker (ed.), *Management of Knee Osteoarthritis in the Younger, Active Patient:*
An Evidence-Based Practical Guide for Clinicians, DOI 10.1007/978-3-662-48530-9_5

suggests that these alterations in articular cartilage can contribute to the development and progression of osteoarthritis [7]. However, the degeneration of normal articular cartilage is not simply the result of ageing and mechanical wear [8]. One needs to be aware of the effect of high-impact and torsional loads, which increase the risk of degeneration of normal joints [6]. This risk is increased in individuals with abnormal joint anatomy, joint instability, disturbances of joint or muscle innervation or inadequate muscle strength or endurance [9]. Although the natural history of cartilage defects is not fully understood, it is generally accepted that they too have the potential to progress to osteoarthritis [10, 11]. Therefore, in considering the aims of cartilage repair and restoration procedures, which are to reduce pain, restore function and limit the onset of osteoarthritis, one must be mindful of the complex pathogenesis that exists in osteoarthritis and, in particular, the challenges that increasing age and altered joint anatomy present.

5.1.2   Evidence-Based Practice

The practice of evidence-based surgery for the management of chondral defects of the knee can be complicated. This is not only due to the heterogeneity in conditions and patients included in studies in the literature but also relates to the regional variation in treatment options approved for use in the clinical setting [12]. However, irrespective of the proposed intervention, a comprehensive understanding of a patient's specific goals, in addition to a discussion of evidence-based management options, is necessary in all cases. Central to this is an understanding of the various described techniques for repair or restoration of articular cartilage defects and an appreciation of the potential complications associated with each [13]. Therefore, the aim of this chapter is to:

I. Describe the surgical treatment options for articular cartilage defects.
II. Provide an up-to-date systematic analysis of the best available evidence for cartilage restoration techniques.

III. Discuss the practical issue of choosing which treatment to use based on resource availability, surgical complexity and cost implications.

5.2   Articular Cartilage Repair and Regeneration Techniques

A variety of treatments have been proposed for articular cartilage defects. The techniques can be broadly classified into marrow stimulation techniques, cellular regeneration and chondral or osteochondral transplantation. Each of these techniques will be discussed briefly with particular focus on the surgical technique, requirement for resources, limitations of the procedure and potential complications.

5.2.1   Marrow Stimulation Techniques

5.2.1.1   Description of Technique
Marrow stimulation techniques include osteochondral drilling [14], abrasion chondroplasty [15] and microfracture [16] (Fig. 5.1). These techniques all seek to stimulate the release of chondroprogenitor cells from the bone cavity through the subchondral plate into the defect to encourage the formation of fibrocartilage (composed of type I and type II collagen)[17]. This layer is unsealed by removing the lower, calcified layer of articular cartilage and by making holes, which penetrate the subchondral plate. They have been performed for more than 45 years beginning with the simple drilling of bony surfaces and burring or 'abrading' the sclerotic lesion and with the use of awls to penetrate eburnated bone to promote blood flow to the bony surface [18].

Microfracture is a technique introduced by Steadman et al., which involves the accurate debridement of all unstable and damaged articular cartilage, down to the subchondral bone plate while maintaining a stable perpendicular edge of healthy cartilage [16]. An arthroscopic awl is used to make multiple holes in the defect 3–4 mm apart, ensuring the subchondral plate is kept

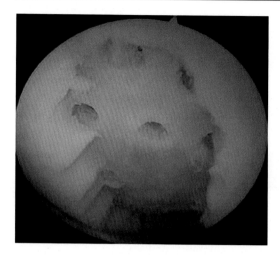

Fig. 5.1 Arthroscopic image of microfracture

intact. The defect is filled with so-called super clot, which is purported to be the optimal environment for pluripotential marrow cells to differentiate into stable tissue (Fig. 5.1) [16]. The rehabilitation protocol is an important part of Steadman's procedure. Early mobility of the joint with continuous passive motion is advocated in conjunction with reduced weight bearing for an extended period.

These techniques are simple and minimally invasive. They can be performed arthroscopically and do not require complex equipment or instrumentation. They are readily available and inexpensive. The advantages of microfracture over drilling might include reduced thermal damage to subchondral bone and the creation of a rougher surface to which repair tissue might adhere more easily. It is also easier to penetrate a defect perpendicularly with a curved awl during an arthroscopic procedure as compared with a drill.

5.2.1.2 Limitations

While often the simplest option for small isolated defects, fibrocartilage is mechanically inferior to hyaline cartilage (composed of type II collagen) [19]. It has also been noted that there is an unpredictable volume of cartilage repair with microfracture [20]. In addition, the failure rates for subsequent cell transplantation are greater in patients that had a prior microfracture. Marrow stimulation techniques have,

therefore, been considered by some to be merely a pain-relieving procedure that at best delays the progression towards osteoarthritis [7, 11].

5.2.1.3 Complications

It has been reported that microfracture can have a significant effect on the micro- and macroarchitecture of subchondral bone [18]. A number of authors have reported subchondral cysts and intralesional osteophytes from 6 months to 5 years postoperatively [21–23]. Recently, it has been postulated that subchondral cyst formation is caused by infiltration of cytokines and metalloproteinases into the subchondral bone subsequent to microfracture [18]. This may explain why the outcome of subsequent cartilage procedures following microfracture has been reported as suboptimal [24].

5.2.1.4 Biological Augmentation of Microfracture

There is increasing evidence that modification or augmentation of microfracture may have the potential to enhance the quality of the repair tissue formed over the cartilage defect and the prospect for improved clinical outcomes [25, 26]. The techniques described seek to provide a biological augment to the microfracture site by delivering cells (i.e. stem cells) and/or individual growth factors (i.e. platelet-rich plasma), with or without the addition of a scaffold material [27–29]. For example, BST-CarGel, a chitosan-based medical device, which is mixed with autologous whole blood and applied to a microfractured cartilage lesion, is thought to physically stabilise the clot and guides and enhances marrow-derived repair [30]; the results of a randomised control trial comparing this treatment to microfracture are discussed later on in the chapter.

5.2.2 Cellular Regeneration Techniques

5.2.2.1 Description of Technique

Cell-based options are used in an attempt to repair hyaline cartilage defects with chondrocyte

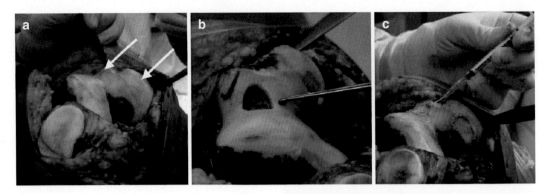

Fig. 5.2 (**a–c**) Operative images of ACI performed to treat cartilage lesions of the trochlea and medial femoral condyle of the right knee: (**a**) two separate full-thickness cartilage lesions (*white arrows*), (**b**) preparation of the defect to the subchondral plate with well-defined edges and (**c**) injection of chondrocytes beneath a collagen patch (Images provided courtesy of Professor David Wood – University of Western Australia)

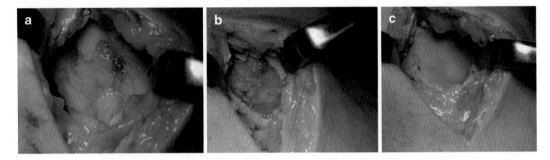

Fig. 5.3 (**a–c**) Operative images of MACI to treat a cartilage lesion on the medial femoral condyle of the left knee: (**a**) medial arthrotomy of the knee demonstrating a full-thickness ulcerated cartilage lesion, (**b**) debridement of the lesion to the subchondral plate and (**c**) insertion of the synthetic matrix to fill the defect (Images provided courtesy of Professor Julian Feller – OrthoSport Victoria)

or stem cell implantation. Autologous chondrocyte implantation (ACI), one of the first applications of cell engineering in orthopaedics, was first performed by Peterson et al. in Gothenburg in 1987 [31]. Cartilage is harvested at an initial arthroscopy, and culture-expanded autologous chondrocyte cells are injected into a chondral defect underneath a patch of periosteum or collagen membrane (Fig. 5.2a–c) [32].

In studies where histological analysis has been performed, it is reported that ACI is capable of producing tissue, which is hyaline-like in some specimens [33]. A variation of the ACI technique using culture-expanded bone marrow stem cells has the advantage of not requiring an additional arthroscopic procedure in order to harvest articular cartilage which has also reported good results [34]. In an attempt to reduce the dedifferentiation of cultured chondrocytes, characterised chondrocyte implantation (CCI) was developed [35]. This technique selects cells with a stable chondrocyte phenotype, which is thought to produce a better quality fill of the defect and enhanced biomechanical properties [35, 36].

Matrix-assisted autologous chondrocyte implantation and related techniques are regarded as second-generation forms of cell implantation that provide a three-dimensional structure for cell adhesion, proliferation and matrix production [37]. A biodegradable type I/III collagen membrane provides a scaffold for cultured autologous chondrocytes, which are seeded onto the surface (Fig. 5.3a–c) [38]. Implantation may be performed arthroscopically or via mini-arthrotomy [39]. Scaffolds are also being used with undifferentiated cell sources, like mesenchymal stem cells derived from bone marrow, synovium and other sources suitable for insertion in a single-stage operative procedure [40–42].

5.2.2.2 Limitations

Although more similar to hyaline cartilage, the best repair tissue achieved as a result of ACI is still not morphologically or histochemically identical to normal hyaline cartilage, and fibrocartilage may be found in a proportion of samples [33]. Whereas some studies have reported that prior bone marrow stimulation and opposing chondral lesions lead to a higher risk of failure, others have shown satisfactory outcomes in both these patient groups [43–46]. Periosteal patch hypertrophy was a significant concern in first-generation ACI, but subsequent generations with enhanced membrane materials have reduced this risk [17]. One of the major drawbacks with ACI, however, is that implantation requires two separate operative procedures with an intervening period of cell culture. This not only creates substantial cost and inconvenience at a clinical level but also adds to the propensity for chondrocytes to dedifferentiate towards a fibroblastic phenotype during culture [47]. Although the literature suggests that procedures using three-dimensional scaffolds are safe, both matrix-assisted autologous chondrocyte implantation and alternative cell-scaffold techniques are still only available for use outside the USA because of variations in their regional regulation [12].

5.2.2.3 Complications

A major proportion of complications after ACI can be summarised by four major diagnoses: symptomatic hypertrophy, disturbed fusion, delamination and graft failure [48]. Among those, the overall complication rate and incidence of hypertrophy of the transplant were higher for periosteal ACI [48]. A systematic review by Harris et al. determined that the failure rate is highest with periosteal ACI and lower with collagen-membrane cover ACI and second-generation techniques [49]. One third of ACI patients underwent a reoperation. Unplanned reoperations were most commonly seen following periosteal ACI, where hypertrophy and

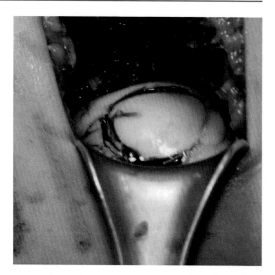

Fig. 5.4 Press-fit allograft using OAT technique to restore the articular congruency of the posterior femoral condyle

delamination were the most frequent complication. Arthrofibrosis was most commonly seen after arthrotomy-based ACI. The use of second-generation techniques and all-arthroscopic techniques reduced the failure, complication and reoperation rate after ACI [49].

5.2.3 Chondral and Osteochondral Transplantation

5.2.3.1 Description of Technique

Osteochondral autologous transplantation (OAT) is a technique that aims to replace the articular cartilage defect with hyaline articular cartilage plugs harvested from elsewhere in the knee (Fig. 5.4) [50]. Osteochondral autograft plugs and mosaicplasty (multiple osteochondral autograft plugs of a smaller diameter) are used to provide a whole osteochondral unit. The advantage of this method of treatment relates to the ability of autogenous bone to integrate more readily compared to cartilage, thus preserving the cartilage-bone interface [51].

Fresh osteochondral allografts may also be used. They are particularly useful for the treatment of larger chondral defects, especially when there is damage to the underlying bone, e.g. cyst formation [52]. Osteochondral allografts are often used for salvage of failed prior cartilage procedures. Off-the-shelf natural or synthetic osteochondral scaffolds that can be impregnated with suitable cells may also be used [53].

Chondral graft is an alternative treatment method, which has come to prominence recently. Minced cartilage autograft and particulated juvenile cartilage allograft have been reported as grafts for chondral repair [54–56]. Histological analysis of both techniques has demonstrated that transplanted cartilage cells migrate from the extracellular matrix, proliferate and form a new hyaline-like cartilage tissue matrix that integrates with the surrounding host tissue. The techniques for minced or particulated grafts are performed in a single-stage procedure and are relatively straightforward. Short-term results have demonstrated that the procedures are safe and effective [56, 57].

5.2.3.2 Limitations

Graft-site mismatch is a potential limitation of osteochondral autograft [58]; grafts may be of different thickness or rotational orientation than the host site and may not be perfectly flush or parallel. Using the mosaicplasty technique may result in gaps. Whereas the bone component of the graft heals, there is no side-to-side healing of the articular layer between the graft and the host. The difference in cartilage thickness and, therefore, mechanical properties of the graft remains a concern [58]. As a result the native biomechanics of the joint may not be recreated. Autograft is also not always feasible for the treatment of large lesions due to the potential for donor site morbidity.

As regards osteochondral allograft, poorer results have been found in older patients, bipolar and patellofemoral lesions and corticosteroid-induced osteonecrosis [59]. Mismatch is also a concern with large allograft, particularly related to the size and depth of the graft and also the contour of the articular surface. Allogenic tissue also has the potential for disease transmission. There is also questionable chondrocyte viability and a lack of integration with surrounding tissue.

The experience with chondral grafting is limited, and given the long-standing belief that integration requires osseous contact, the long-term survival and integration of the graft with host tissue requires further study. Synthetic osteochondral plugs are a very attractive treatment option; however, the stringent regulatory processes required for approval of this technology are extremely challenging not to mention costly. It has been estimated that it may cost up to $500 million to bring a new biological option to the market in the USA [12].

5.2.3.3 Complications

Despite the maintenance of the integrity of osteochondral autograft plug following transfer, the surround articular cartilage can continue to deteriorate, leading to a wide area of further chondral damage [50]. Graft delamination has been reported with osteochondral grafting and also with particulated cartilage grafting [54, 60]. Articular surface incongruity and failure of osseous incorporation can also occur following osteochondral grafting, which is best appreciated on postoperative MRI [60]. Osteochondral allografts are also capable of causing *kissing lesions* on the tibial plateau if left too proud on the femoral condyle [61]. Recent studies on a biphasic synthetic plug have presented concerning findings with respect to both clinical outcomes and structural analysis, with the finding of fibrous tissue repair and foreign-body giant cells at the defect site at the time of revision surgery [53].

5.3 Evidence-Based Practice

Despite an increase in research focus on the treatment techniques available for articular cartilage defects of the knee, there remains no consensus as to the best available treatment option [62]. Furthermore, the vast majority of these studies have been of low methodological quality; only 9 % of 194 studies on cartilage treatment were level I randomised controlled trials [63] with the majority (76 %) being level IV evidence.

For the purpose of providing clarity on the best available evidence in the literature, a review of the systematic reviews is provided in this chapter along with an up-to-date systematic review of all level I studies performed to assess the outcome of a variety of cartilage repair and regeneration techniques.

5.3.1 Review of Systematic Reviews

Eighteen systematic reviews have been identified which focus on a variety of articular cartilage treatment techniques (Table 5.1). As with any systematic review, the evidence provided is only as good as the original studies chosen as part of the selection process. Only two studies provided a review of level I evidence [72, 76]. Vasiliadis et al., in their study, determined that there was insufficient evidence available from level I studies to support ACI over OAT, MACI or microfracture. Moreover, Bekker et al. could only identify four level I evidence studies published between 2003 and 2008 [76]. The authors concluded that smaller lesions should be treated by microfracture or single plug OAT and that ACI or OAT resulted in improved outcomes in active patients with large articular cartilage lesions compared to microfracture.

A further five systematic reviews contain both level I and level II evidence. Of these systematic reviews, two found that there was insufficient evidence to determine a superior treatment between ACI, OAT and microfracture [71, 77]. The remaining three studies provided differing conclusions; Lynch et al., comparing OAT with microfracture and ACI, concluded that OAT is effective in smaller lesions ($<2 \text{ cm}^2$), but ACI has superior long-term results, albeit the latter conclusion was based on the results of a single randomised control conducted by Bentley et al. in 2012 [58, 79]; Goyal et al., in their comparison of microfracture versus CCI, ACI and OAT, reported that microfracture has good clinical outcomes in small lesions and lower-demand patients; however, treatment failures were identified at 5–10 years [67]; finally, Harris et al., comparing ACI with OAT and microfracture, stated that ACI was associated with improved outcomes in defects $>4 \text{ cm}^2$ and ACI and OAT gave comparable short-term results [80]. Interestingly, these studies were all carried out over a period of 5 years, which emphasises the need to be cautious in reading too much into systematic reviews as very similar data can be interpreted quite differently.

Thirteen further systematic reviews were analysed. Three studies contained a review of only level IV evidence [64, 69, 70]. In two of these three studies, only one technique was studied, and unsurprisingly, the results demonstrated favourable outcomes. The third study by Windt et al. focused on all cartilage treatment techniques in the setting of early osteoarthritis and determined that ACI could provide good short- to medium-term outcomes. Of the remaining eight articles, the level of evidence ranged from level I to IV; six out of these eight studies determined that there was insufficient evidence to determine superiority for any of techniques assessed, thus providing little clarity on the dilemma of which articular cartilage treatment to use.

5.3.2 Level I Evidence: An Up-to-Date Systematic Review

For the purpose of this chapter, an up-to-date systematic review was performed of only level I studies according to PRISMA guidelines (Fig. 5.5). The studies included in this systematic review were all randomised controlled trials of a variety of articular treatment techniques, representing the most widely accepted practices internationally, with both short- and long-term results being reported. Studies were only selected if they met exacting methodological criteria and had a low risk of bias. Nine studies were identified with the highest level of clinical evidence from the current body of research on the surgical treatment of articular cartilage lesions of the knee (Table 5.2). The main finding was that regardless of the type of cartilage regeneration technique used, an improvement in the measured clinical outcome was observed compared to pre-surgical baseline levels. In the majority of trials (7/9), microfracture was used as the control group. Although clinical outcomes varied between studies, microfracture was found to be either equivalent or inferior to OAT, ACI and MACI, but never superior. No significant difference was found between the failure rates of various techniques in any trial up to 5 years. However, as expected, failure rates increased with time, and a significant difference could be detected between treatment methods after 10 years, emphasising the importance of long-term follow-up (Table 5.3). Lesion size was determined to be important with the overall results of the systematic

Table 5.1 A review of systematic reviews

Author	Year	Number of studies	Systematic review	Comparative treatments	Level of evidence	Clinical outcome
De Caro et al. [64]	2015	11	Fresh osteochondral allograft		Level IV	Good long-term result with fresh osteochondral allograft. Procedure burdened by cost and access to grafts
Kon et al. [65]	2015	127	Scaffolds with and without cells	Clinical setting – cells and no cells	Levels I–IV	Good short-term outcome with scaffolds with and without cells
Lynch et al. [58]	2015	9	OAT	MF, ACI	Levels I–II	OAT effective in smaller lesions (<2 cm^2). Known risk of failure at 2–4 years
Oussedik et al. [66]	2015	34	MF or ACI	CCI, MACI	Levels I–IV	MF effective in smaller lesions, MACI more effective than MF, ACI an effective treatment
Goyal et al. [67]	2013	15	MF	ACI, CCI, OAT	Levels I–II	MF had good clinical outcomes in small lesions and lower-demand patients. Treatment failures identified at 5–10 years
Filardo et al. [68]	2013	18	MSC		Levels III–IV	Insufficient evidence
Filardo et al. [62]	2013	51	Scaffold-based repair		Levels I–IV	Insufficient evidence
De Windt et al. [69]	2013	9	All treatments in the setting of early OA	ACI, CF, MF	Level IV	ACI could provide good short- to medium-term clinical outcomes in the setting of early OA
Chahal et al. [70]	2013	14	OAT		Level IV	Favourable outcomes and high satisfaction rates at intermediate follow-up
Vavken et al. [71]	2010	9	ACI	MF, OAT	Levels I–II	Insufficient evidence
Vasiliadis et al. [72]	2010	6	ACI	OAT, MACI, MF	Level I	Insufficient evidence
Harris et al. [73]	2010	13	ACI	OAT, MF	Levels I–II	ACI associated with improved outcomes in defects >4 cm^2. ACI and OAT gave comparable short-term results
Nakamura et al. [74]	2009	39	Cell-based therapy	ACI, CCI, MACI	Levels I–IV	Insufficient evidence
Mithoefer et al. [20]	2009	28	MF		Levels I–IV	MF has effective short-term outcomes
Kon et al. [75]	2009	18	MACI		Levels I–IV	Insufficient evidence
Bekkers et al. [76]	2009	4	All treatments	ACI, CCI, MF, OAT	Level I	MF had good results with <2.5 cm^2 lesions, ACI or OAT superior if lesion >2.5 cm^2. Active patients have better results with OAT or ACI
Magnussen et al. [77]	2008	6	All treatments	ACI, MACI, MF, OAT	Levels I–II	No technique was superior
Ruano-Ravina and Diaz [78]	2006	9	ACI	MF, OAT	Levels I–IV	No evidence of superiority of ACI

Key: *C* carbon fibres, *MF* microfracture, *CCI* characterised chondrocyte implantation, *ACI* autologous chondrocyte implantation, *OAT* osteochondral autologous transplantation, *MSC* mesenchymal stem cell

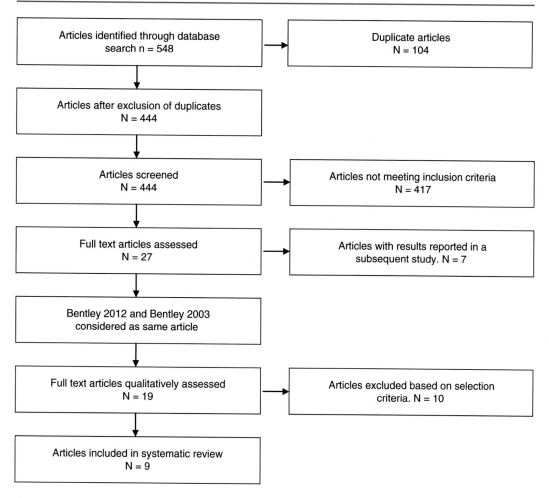

Fig. 5.5 PRISMA flowchart for systematic review of level I studies

Table 5.2 Cartilage technique failure rate in level I studies

	Follow-up	Treatment	Failure	Significant difference
Bartlett et al. [81]	1 year	ACI	0	NS
		MACI	2 of 47 (4 %)	
Bentley et al. [79]	10 years	ACI	10 of 58 (17 %)	$P < 0.001$
		OAT	23 of 42 (55 %)	
Gudas et al. [82]	10 years	OAT	4 (14 %)	$P < 0.05$
		Microfracture	11 (38 %)	
Gudas et al. [83]	3 years	–	Not stated	–
Knutsen et al. [23]	5 years	ACI	9 (mean 26.2 months)	NS
		Microfracture	9 (mean 37.8 months)	$(P = 0.101)$
Saris et al. [84]	2 years	MACI	0	NS
		Microfracture	2	
Stanish et al. [30]	1 year	–	Not stated	–
Ulstein et al. [85]	9.8 years	Microfracture	6 (54 %)	NS
		OAT	5 (36 %)	
Vanlauwe et al. [35]	5 years	CCI	7 (13.7 %)	NS
		Microfracture	10 (16.4 %)	$(P = 0.561)$

Table 5.3 Clinical outcomes summary

	Follow up	ICRS [11]	Tegner [86]	KOOS [87]	SF-36/SF-12 [88] PCS	SF-36/SF-12 [88] MCS	WOMAC [89]	IKDC subjective [90]	Lysholm [91, 92]	Cincinnati [93]	EQ 5D [94]	Stanmore functional rating	VAS
Microfracture vs OAT													
Gudas et al. [82]	10 years	↑OATS	↑OATS	–	–	–	–	–	–	–	–	–	–
Gudas et al. [83]	3 years	–	↑OATS[d]	–	–	–	–	↑OATS[d]	–	–	–	–	–
Ulstein et al. [85]	9.8 years	–	–	NS	–	–	–	–	NS	–	–	–	–
Microfracture vs ACI or MACI													
Knutsen et al. [23]	5 years	–	NS	–	NS	–	–	–	NS	–	–	–	NS
Saris et al. [84]	2 years	–	–	↑MACI	↑MACI	NS	–	NS	–	↑MACI[a]	NS	–	–
Vanlauwe et al. [35]	5 years	–	–	NS[b]	–	–	–	–	–	–	–	–	–
Microfracture vs BST-CarGel													
Stanish et al. [30]	1 year	–	–	–	NS	NS	NS	–	–	–	–	–	–
OAT vs ACI													
Bentley et al. [95]	19 months	–	–	–	–	–	–	–	–	NS[c]	–	NS	–
ACI vs MACI													
Bartlett et al. [81]	1 year	–	–	–	–	–	–	–	–	NS[a]	–	NS	NS

[a]Modified cincinnati scoring system used

[b]Change from baseline scores used, overall results were non significant. CCI group had improvement with symptoms under 3 years

[c]Cincinnati rating score, overall results were non significant. ACI group had better score for MFC lesions

[d]Concomitant anterior cruciate ligament reconstruction

ICRS International cartilage repair society; *KOOS* knee injury and osteoarthritis outcome score; *SF-36/SF-12* short form 36 or 12; *WOMAC* Western Ontario and McMaster universities osteoarthritis index; *IKDC* International knee documentation committee; *EQ 5D* European quality of life; *Stanmore* stanmore functional rating; *VAS* visual analogue score review suggesting improved short-term results with cartilage regeneration techniques (OAT, ACI and MACI) over MF in larger lesions (>4.5 cm²)[23, 79, 81, 84].

A systematic review of high-quality randomised controlled trials comparing cartilage repair techniques was unable to ascertain the most effective treatment method. However, it did determine that regardless of the type of cartilage regeneration technique used, an improvement in the measured clinical outcome was observed compared to pre-surgical baseline levels and microfracture demonstrated comparable but not superior clinical outcomes to OAT and cartilage regenerative techniques. Treatment of larger articular defects (>4.5 cm²) with OAT or ACI resulted in improved clinical outcomes over microfracture. Given that no significant difference in failure rates could be detected up to a period of 5 years, it is important that future studies be followed to at least this term before definitive conclusions can be made on treatment efficacy.

5.4   Cost-Effectiveness of Treatment

It is evident from the fact that microfracture is used for the control in the majority of studies that it is still considered the gold standard treatment for cartilage defects of the knee. In order to frame the decision-making process about which cartilage treatment method to use, one must first consider the potential advantages of microfracture such as low cost, single-stage procedure, readily available and no donor morbidity. In the age of escalating healthcare costs, the challenge exists for other treatments to prove their superiority not just in the short term but also in the longer term to justify their expense and technical complexity.

Considering the high cost associated with engineering chondrocytes and osteochondral grafting techniques with equivocal clinical data, there are limited studies focusing on the cost-effectiveness of these therapies. While Clar et al. attempted a cost-comparison analysis in their systematic review of four RCTs in 2005, they were unable to generate conclusions due to lim-

ited evidence [96]. They state that the quality-of-life gain of ACI would need to be 70–100 % greater than microfracture over 2 years, or alternatively 10–20 % maintained over 10 years, to justify the use of ACI.

Samuelson et al. in 2012 carried out a cost-analysis using a decision analysis model based on outcome data, and complication rates from patients undergoing ACI were derived from the best evidence in the literature [97]. They determined that both periosteal ACI and collagen patch ACI were both cost-effective. Interestingly, the quoted price of treatment was $66,752 for periosteal ACI and $66,939.50 for collagen patch ACI. The conclusion of this study would be in keeping with an earlier study by Minas et al. in which the authors stated that ACI remained cost-effective even when outcomes were less than optimal [98]. Frappier et al. have also claimed that the superior results of BST-CarGel as an adjunct to microfracture compared to microfracture alone potentially represent a cost-saving alternative for patients with knee cartilage injury by reducing the risk of clinical events through regeneration of chondral tissue with hyaline characteristics [99]. However, as has been determined the *best evidence* in the literature offers quite variable results with respect to the quality of cartilage tissue produced, associated complications and particularly long-term outcomes, which may have a significant effect on these analyses. Therefore, the cost-effectiveness in favour of ACI or other alternative treatments (BST-CarGel) at best remains controversial and certainly inconclusive when considered on a global stage.

Conclusion
Despite the growing interest in the area of cartilage regeneration in recent years, the generally low methodological quality of studies means that results need to be interpreted with extreme caution [63]. At present, orthopaedic surgeons treating cartilage lesions of the knee still debride the articular surface and penetrate the subchondral plate with the intention of decreasing symptoms and restoring or maintaining a functional articular surface. Oftentimes, this is done in the knowledge that

the results of these procedures vary considerably among patients.

While experimental studies have revealed success with a wide variety of treatment techniques to stimulate the formation of a new articular surface, thus far none of these methods have been able to reliably prevent the onset of osteoarthritis. What is increasingly evident is that a holistic approach needs to be adopted for the treatment of cartilage lesions in the knee, with due consideration given to the structural and functional abnormalities of the involved joint and, importantly, the patient's expectations for future use of the joint. If evidence based has taught us anything about the treatment of cartilage lesion, it is that *nothing ruins results like follow-up*. Evidence in the literature should not be adopted with blind faith. Assessment of which specific technique to use should be made on an individual case-by-case basis, bearing in mind the technical skills and resources required, the availability of the technology and the needs of the patient. It is important that future studies be followed out to at least 5 years before definitive conclusions can be made on treatment efficacy.

References

1. Pearle AD, Warren RF, Rodeo SA. Basic science of articular cartilage and osteoarthritis. Clin Sports Med. 2005;24(1):1–12.
2. Heir S, Nerhus TK, Rotterud JH, Loken S, Ekeland A, Engebretsen L, et al. Focal cartilage defects in the knee impair quality of life as much as severe osteoarthritis: a comparison of knee injury and osteoarthritis outcome score in 4 patient categories scheduled for knee surgery. Am J Sports Med. 2010;38(2):231–7.
3. Gomoll AH, Farr J, Gillogly SD, Kercher J, Minas T. Surgical management of articular cartilage defects of the knee. J Bone Joint Surg Am. 2010;92(14):2470–90.
4. Cole BJ, Pascual-Garrido C, Grumet RC. Surgical management of articular cartilage defects in the knee. J Bone Joint Surg Am. 2009;91(7):1778–90.
5. Bertrand J, Cromme C, Umlauf D, Frank S, Pap T. Molecular mechanisms of cartilage remodelling in osteoarthritis. Int J Biochem Cell Biol. 2010;42(10):1594–601.
6. Buckwalter JA, Mankin HJ. Articular cartilage: degeneration and osteoarthritis, repair, regeneration, and transplantation. Instr Course Lect. 1998;47:487–504.
7. He Y, Siebuhr AS, Brandt-Hansen NU, Wang J, Su D, Zheng Q, et al. Type X collagen levels are elevated in serum from human osteoarthritis patients and associated with biomarkers of cartilage degradation and inflammation. BMC Musculoskelet Disord. 2014;15:309.
8. Buckwalter JA. Articular cartilage injuries. Clin Orthop Relat Res. 2002;402:21–37.
9. Buckwalter JA. Articular cartilage: injuries and potential for healing. J Orthop Sports Phys Ther. 1998;28(4):192–202.
10. Alford JW, Cole BJ. Cartilage restoration, part 1: basic science, historical perspective, patient evaluation, and treatment options. Am J Sports Med. 2005; 33(2):295–306.
11. Brittberg M, Winalski CS. Evaluation of cartilage injuries and repair. J Bone Joint Surg Am. 2003;85-A Suppl 2:58–69.
12. Moran CJ, Pascual-Garrido C, Chubinskaya S, Potter HG, Warren RF, Cole BJ, et al. Restoration of articular cartilage. J Bone Joint Surg A. 2014;96(4):336–44.
13. Mithoefer K, Della Villa S. Return to sports after articular cartilage repair in the football (soccer) player. Cartilage. 2012;3(1 Suppl):57s–62.
14. Schmidt H, Schulze KJ, Cyffka R. Results of treatment of cartilage damage by Pridie drilling of the knee joint. Beitr Orthop Traumatol. 1988;35(3):117–22.
15. Johnson LL. Arthroscopic abrasion arthroplasty historical and pathologic perspective: present status. Arthroscopy. 1986;2(1):54–69.
16. Steadman JR, Rodkey WG, Rodrigo JJ. Microfracture: surgical technique and rehabilitation to treat chondral defects. Clin Orthop Relat Res. 2001;(391 Suppl): S362–9.
17. Mollon B, Kandel R, Chahal J, Theodoropoulos J. The clinical status of cartilage tissue regeneration in humans. Osteoarthritis Cartilage. 2013;21(12):1824–33.
18. Bert JM. Abandoning microfracture of the knee: has the time come? Arthroscopy. 2015;31(3):501–5.
19. Franke O, Durst K, Maier V, Goken M, Birkholz T, Schneider H, et al. Mechanical properties of hyaline and repair cartilage studied by nanoindentation. Acta Biomater. 2007;3(6):873–81.
20. Mithoefer K, McAdams T, Williams RJ, Kreuz PC, Mandelbaum BR. Clinical efficacy of the microfracture technique for articular cartilage repair in the knee: an evidence-based systematic analysis. Am J Sports Med. 2009;37(10):2053–63.
21. Orth P, Goebel L, Wolfram U, Ong MF, Graber S, Kohn D, et al. Effect of subchondral drilling on the microarchitecture of subchondral bone: analysis in a large animal model at 6 months. Am J Sports Med. 2012;40(4):828–36.
22. Gudas R, Simonaityte R, Cekanauskas E, Tamosiunas R. A prospective, randomized clinical study of osteochondral autologous transplantation versus microfracture for the treatment of osteochondritis dissecans in the knee joint in children. J Pediatr Orthop. 2009; 29(7):741–8.

23. Knutsen G, Drogset JO, Engebretsen L, Grontvedt T, Isaksen V, Ludvigsen TC, et al. A randomized trial comparing autologous chondrocyte implantation with microfracture. Findings at five years. J Bone Joint Surg Am Vol. 2007;89(10):2105–12.
24. Jungmann PM, Salzmann GM, Schmal H, Pestka JM, Sudkamp NP, Niemeyer P. Autologous chondrocyte implantation for treatment of cartilage defects of the knee: what predicts the need for reintervention? Am J Sports Med. 2012;40(1):58–67.
25. Farr J, Cole B, Dhawan A, Kercher J, Sherman S. Clinical cartilage restoration: evolution and overview. Clin Orthop Relat Res. 2011;469(10): 2696–705.
26. Chen H, Sun J, Hoemann CD, Lascau-Coman V, Ouyang W, McKee MD, et al. Drilling and microfracture lead to different bone structure and necrosis during bone-marrow stimulation for cartilage repair. J Orthop Res. 2009;27(11):1432–8.
27. Fortier LA, Barker JU, Strauss EJ, McCarrel TM, Cole BJ. The role of growth factors in cartilage repair. Clin Orthop Relat Res. 2011;469(10):2706–15.
28. Fortier LA, Potter HG, Rickey EJ, Schnabel LV, Foo LF, Chong LR, et al. Concentrated bone marrow aspirate improves full-thickness cartilage repair compared with microfracture in the equine model. J Bone Joint Surg Am. 2010;92(10):1927–37.
29. Sermer C, Devitt B, Chahal J, Kandel R, Theodoropoulos J. The addition of platelet-rich plasma to scaffolds used for cartilage repair: a review of human and animal studies. Arthroscopy. 2015; 31(8):1607–25.
30. Stanish WD, McCormack R, Forriol F, Mohtadi N, Pelet S, Desnoyers J, et al. Novel scaffold-based BST-CarGel treatment results in superior cartilage repair compared with microfracture in a randomized controlled trial. J Bone Joint Surg Am Vol. 2013; 95(18):1640–50.
31. Peterson L, Minas T, Brittberg M, Nilsson A, Sjogren-Jansson E, Lindahl A. Two- to 9-year outcome after autologous chondrocyte transplantation of the knee. Clin Orthop Relat Res. 2000;374:212–34.
32. Brittberg M, Lindahl A, Nilsson A, Ohlsson C, Isaksson O, Peterson L. Treatment of deep cartilage defects in the knee with autologous chondrocyte transplantation. N Engl J Med. 1994;331(14): 889–95.
33. Roberts S, McCall IW, Darby AJ, Menage J, Evans H, Harrison PE, et al. Autologous chondrocyte implantation for cartilage repair: monitoring its success by magnetic resonance imaging and histology. Arthritis Res Ther. 2003;5(1):R60–73.
34. Wakitani S. Repair of articular cartilage defect by cell transplantation. J Artif Organs. 2000;3(2):98–101.
35. Vanlauwe J, Saris DB, Victor J, Almqvist KF, Bellemans J, Luyten FP, et al. Five-year outcome of characterized chondrocyte implantation versus microfracture for symptomatic cartilage defects of the knee: early treatment matters. Am J Sports Med. 2011; 39(12):2566–74.

36. Dhollander AA, Verdonk PC, Lambrecht S, Verdonk R, Elewaut D, Verbruggen G, et al. Short-term outcome of the second generation characterized chondrocyte implantation for the treatment of cartilage lesions in the knee. Knee Surg Sports Traumatol Arthrosc. 2012;20(6):1118–27.
37. Kon E, Filardo G, Di Martino A, Marcacci M. ACI and MACI. J Knee Surg. 2012;25(1):17–22.
38. Kon E, Delcogliano M, Filardo G, Montaperto C, Marcacci M. Second generation issues in cartilage repair. Sports Med Arthrosc Rev. 2008;16(4):221–9.
39. Kon E, Filardo G, Di Martino A, Patella S, D'Orazio L, Marcacci M. Arthroscopic autologous chondrocyte transplantation – prospective study: results at minimum 7 years follow-up. Arthroscopy. 2011;1:e181–2.
40. Fan J, Varshney RR, Ren L, Cai D, Wang DA. Synovium-derived mesenchymal stem cells: a new cell source for musculoskeletal regeneration. Tissue Eng Part B Rev. 2009;15(1):75–86.
41. Haleem AM, Singergy AA, Sabry D, Atta HM, Rashed LA, Chu CR, et al. The clinical use of human culture-expanded autologous bone marrow mesenchymal stem cells transplanted on platelet-rich fibrin glue in the treatment of articular cartilage defects: a pilot study and preliminary results. Cartilage. 2010;1(4):253–61.
42. Evans CH. Barriers to the clinical translation of orthopedic tissue engineering. Tissue Eng Part B Rev. 2011;17(6):437–41.
43. Minas T, Gomoll AH, Rosenberger R, Royce RO, Bryant T. Increased failure rate of autologous chondrocyte implantation after previous treatment with marrow stimulation techniques. Am J Sports Med. 2009;37(5):902–8.
44. Minas T, Gomoll AH, Solhpour S, Rosenberger R, Probst C, Bryant T. Autologous chondrocyte implantation for joint preservation in patients with early osteoarthritis. Clin Orthop Relat Res. 2010;468(1): 147–57.
45. Rosenberger RE, Gomoll AH, Bryant T, Minas T. Repair of large chondral defects of the knee with autologous chondrocyte implantation in patients 45 years or older. Am J Sports Med. 2008;36(12): 2336–44.
46. Pascual-Garrido C, Slabaugh MA, L'Heureux DR, Friel NA, Cole BJ. Recommendations and treatment outcomes for patellofemoral articular cartilage defects with autologous chondrocyte implantation: prospective evaluation at average 4-year follow-up. Am J Sports Med. 2009;37 Suppl 1:33S–41.
47. Smith GD, Knutsen G, Richardson JB. A clinical review of cartilage repair techniques. J Bone Joint Surg Br Vol. 2005;87(4):445–9.
48. Niemeyer P, Pestka JM, Kreuz PC, Erggelet C, Schmal H, Suedkamp NP, et al. Characteristic complications after autologous chondrocyte implantation for cartilage defects of the knee joint. Am J Sports Med. 2008;36(11):2091–9.
49. Harris JD, Siston RA, Brophy RH, Lattermann C, Carey JL, Flanigan DC. Failures, re-operations, and

complications after autologous chondrocyte implantation: a systematic review (structured abstract). Osteoarthritis Cartilage [Internet]. 2011;19(7):779–91.

50. Bobic V. Arthroscopic osteochondral autograft transplantation in anterior cruciate ligament reconstruction: a preliminary clinical study. Knee Surg Sports Traumatol Arthrosc. 1996;3(4):262–4.

51. Krych AJ, Harnly HW, Rodeo SA, Williams 3rd RJ. Activity levels are higher after osteochondral autograft transfer mosaicplasty than after microfracture for articular cartilage defects of the knee: a retrospective comparative study. J Bone Joint Surg Am. 2012;94(11):971–8.

52. Demange M, Gomoll AH. The use of osteochondral allografts in the management of cartilage defects. Curr Rev Musculoskelet Med. 2012;5(3):229–35.

53. Dhollander AA, Liekens K, Almqvist KF, Verdonk R, Lambrecht S, Elewaut D, et al. A pilot study of the use of an osteochondral scaffold plug for cartilage repair in the knee and how to deal with early clinical failures. Arthroscopy. 2012;28(2):225–33.

54. Farr J, Cole BJ, Sherman S, Karas V. Particulated articular cartilage: CAIS and DeNovo NT. J Knee Surg. 2012;25(1):23–9.

55. Cole BJ, Farr J, Winalski CS, Hosea T, Richmond J, Mandelbaum B, et al. Outcomes after a single-stage procedure for cell-based cartilage repair: a prospective clinical safety trial with 2-year follow-up. Am J Sports Med [Internet]. 2011;39(6):1170–9.

56. Farr J, Tabet SK, Margerrison E, Cole BJ. Clinical, radiographic, and histological outcomes after cartilage repair with particulated juvenile articular cartilage: a 2-year prospective study. Am J Sports Med. 2014;42(6):1417–25.

57. Cole BJ, DeBerardino T, Brewster R, Farr J, Levine DW, Nissen C, et al. Outcomes of autologous chondrocyte implantation in study of the treatment of articular repair (STAR) patients with osteochondritis dissecans. Am J Sports Med. 2012;40(9):2015–22.

58. Lynch TS, Patel RM, Benedick A, Amin NH, Jones MH, Miniaci A. Systematic review of autogenous osteochondral transplant outcomes. Arthroscopy. 2015;31(4):746–54.

59. Levy YD, Gortz S, Pulido PA, McCauley JC, Bugbee WD. Do fresh osteochondral allografts successfully treat femoral condyle lesions? Clin Orthop Relat Res. 2013;471(1):231–7.

60. Trattnig S, Millington SA, Szomolanyi P, Marlovits S. MR imaging of osteochondral grafts and autologous chondrocyte implantation. Eur Radiol. 2007; 17(1):103–18.

61. Johnson MR, LaPrade RF. Tibial plateau "Kissing Lesion" from a proud osteochondral autograft. Am J Orthop. 2011;40(7):359–61.

62. Filardo G, Kon E, Roffi A, Di Martino A, Marcacci M. Scaffold-based repair for cartilage healing: a systematic review and technical note. Arthroscopy. 2013;29(1):174–86.

63. Harris JD, Erickson BJ, Abrams GD, Cvetanovich GL, McCormick FM, Gupta AK, et al. Methodologic quality of knee articular cartilage studies. Arthroscopy. 2013;29(7):1243–52.e5.

64. De Caro F, Bisicchia S, Amendola A, Ding L. Large fresh osteochondral allografts of the knee: a systematic clinical and basic science review of the literature. Arthroscopy. 2015;31(4):757–65.

65. Kon E, Roffi A, Filardo G, Tesei G, Marcacci M. Scaffold-based cartilage treatments: with or without cells? A systematic review of preclinical and clinical evidence. Arthroscopy. 2015;31(4):767–75.

66. Oussedik S, Tsitskaris K, Parker D. Treatment of articular cartilage lesions of the knee by microfracture or autologous chondrocyte implantation: a systematic review. Arthroscopy. 2015;31(4):732–44.

67. Goyal D, Keyhani S, Lee EH, Hui JHP. Evidence-based status of microfracture technique: a systematic review of level I and II studies. Arthroscopy. 2013; 29(9):1579–88.

68. Filardo G, Madry H, Jelic M, Roffi A, Cucchiarini M, Kon E. Mesenchymal stem cells for the treatment of cartilage lesions: from preclinical findings to clinical application in orthopaedics. Knee Surg Sports Traumatol Arthrosc. 2013;21(8):1717–29.

69. de Windt TS, Vonk LA, Brittberg M, Saris DBF. Treatment and prevention of (early) osteoarthritis using articular cartilage repair-fact or fiction? A systematic review. Cartilage. 2013;4(3 Suppl):5S–12.

70. Chahal J, Gross AE, Gross C, Mall N, Dwyer T, Chahal A, et al. Outcomes of osteochondral allograft transplantation in the knee. Arthroscopy. 2013;29(3): 575–88.

71. Vavken P, Samartzis D. Effectiveness of autologous chondrocyte implantation in cartilage repair of the knee: a systematic review of controlled trials. Osteoarthritis Cartilage. 2010;18(6):857–63.

72. Vasiliadis Haris S, Wasiak J. Autologous chondrocyte implantation for full thickness articular cartilage defects of the knee. Cochrane Database Syst Rev [Internet]. 2010;(10):CD003323.

73. Harris JD, Siston RA, Pan X, Flanigan DC. Autologous chondrocyte implantation: a systematic review (provisional abstract). J Bone Joint Surg Am Vol [Internet]. 2010;92(12):2220–33.

74. Nakamura N, Miyama T, Engebretsen L, Yoshikawa H, Shino K. Cell-based therapy in articular cartilage lesions of the knee. Arthroscopy. 2009;25(5):531–52.

75. Kon E, Verdonk P, Condello V, Delcogliano M, Dhollander A, Filardo G, et al. Matrix-assisted autologous chondrocyte transplantation for the repair of cartilage defects of the knee: systematic clinical data review and study quality analysis. Am J Sports Med. 2009;37 Suppl 1:156S–66.

76. Bekkers JE, Inklaar M, Saris DB. Treatment selection in articular cartilage lesions of the knee: a systematic review. Am J Sports Med. 2009;37 Suppl 1:148S–55.

77. Magnussen RA, Dunn WR, Carey JL, Spindler KP. Treatment of focal articular cartilage defects in the knee: a systematic review (structured abstract). Clin Orthop Relat Res [Internet]. 2008;466(4): 952–62.

78. Ruano-Ravina A, Diaz MJ. Autologous chondrocyte implantation: a systematic review. Osteoarthritis Cartilage. 2006;14(1):47–51.

79. Bentley G, Biant LC, Vijayan S, Macmull S, Skinner JA, Carrington RWJ. Minimum ten-year results of a prospective randomised study of autologous chondrocyte implantation versus mosaicplasty for symptomatic articular cartilage lesions of the knee. J Bone Joint Surg Br Vol [Internet]. 2012;94 B(4):504–9.

80. Harris JD, Brophy RH, Siston RA, Flanigan DC. Systematic review: treatment of chondral defects in the athlete's knee (provisional abstract). Arthroscopy [Internet]. 2010;26(6):841–52.

81. Bartlett W, Flanagan AM, Gooding CR, Skinner JA, Carrington RW, Briggs TW, et al. Autologous chondrocyte implantation versus matrix-induced autologous chondrocyte implantation for osteochondral defects of the knee: a prospective, randomised study. J Bone Joint Surg Br Vol [Internet]. 2005; 87(5):640–5.

82. Gudas R, Gudaite A, Pocius A, Gudiene A, Cekanauskas E, Monastyreckiene E, et al. Ten-year follow-up of a prospective, randomized clinical study of mosaic osteochondral autologous transplantation versus microfracture for the treatment of osteochondral defects in the knee joint of athletes. Am J Sports Med. 2012;40(11):2499–508.

83. Gudas R, Gudaite A, Mickevicius T, Masiulis N, Simonaityte R, Cekanauskas E, et al. Comparison of osteochondral autologous transplantation, microfracture, or debridement techniques in articular cartilage lesions associated with anterior cruciate ligament injury: a prospective study with a 3-year follow-up. Arthroscopy. 2013;29(1):89–97.

84. Saris D, Price A, Widuchowski W, Bertrand-Marchand M, Caron J, Drogset JO, et al. Matrix-applied characterized autologous cultured chondrocytes versus microfracture: two-year follow-up of a prospective randomized trial. Am J Sports Med. 2014;42(6):1384–94.

85. Ulstein S, Aroen A, Rotterud JH, Loken S, Engebretsen L, Heir S. Microfracture technique versus osteochondral autologous transplantation mosaicplasty in patients with articular chondral lesions of the knee: a prospective randomized trial with long-term follow-up. Knee Surg Sports Traumatol Arthrosc [Internet]. 2014;22(6):1207–15.

86. Tegner Y, Lysholm J. Rating systems in the evaluation of knee ligament injuries. Clin Orthop Relat Res. 1985;198:43–9.

87. Roos EM, Roos HP, Lohmander LS, Ekdahl C, Beynnon BD. Knee injury and osteoarthritis outcome score (KOOS) – development of a self-administered outcome measure. J Orthop Sports Phys Ther. 1998;28(2):88–96.

88. Ware Jr JE, Sherbourne CD. The MOS 36-item short-form health survey (SF-36). I. Conceptual framework and item selection. Med Care. 1992;30(6):473–83.

89. Bellamy N, Buchanan WW, Goldsmith CH, Campbell J, Stitt LW. Validation study of WOMAC: a health status instrument for measuring clinically important patient relevant outcomes to antirheumatic drug therapy in patients with osteoarthritis of the hip or knee. J Rheumatol. 1988;15(12):1833–40.

90. Irrgang JJ, Anderson AF, Boland AL, Harner CD, Kurosaka M, Neyret P, et al. Development and validation of the international knee documentation committee subjective knee form. Am J Sports Med. 2001; 29(5):600–13.

91. Kocher MS, Steadman JR, Briggs KK, Sterett WI, Hawkins RJ. Reliability, validity, and responsiveness of the Lysholm knee scale for various chondral disorders of the knee. J Bone Joint Surg Am. 2004; 86-A(6):1139–45.

92. Lysholm J, Gillquist J. Evaluation of knee ligament surgery results with special emphasis on use of a scoring scale. Am J Sports Med. 1982;10(3):150–4.

93. Barber-Westin SD, Noyes FR, McCloskey JW. Rigorous statistical reliability, validity, and responsiveness testing of the Cincinnati knee rating system in 350 subjects with uninjured, injured, or anterior cruciate ligament-reconstructed knees. Am J Sports Med. 1999;27(4):402–16.

94. EuroQol G. EuroQol – a new facility for the measurement of health-related quality of life. Health Policy. 1990;16(3):199–208.

95. Bentley G, Biant LC, Carrington RWJ, Akmal M, Goldberg A, Williams AM, et al. A prospective, randomised comparison of autologous chondrocyte implantation versus mosaicplasty for osteochondral defects in the knee. J Bone Joint Surg B. 2003;85(2):223–30.

96. Clar C, Cummins E, McIntyre L, Thomas S, Lamb J, Bain L, et al. Clinical and cost-effectiveness of autologous chondrocyte implantation for cartilage defects in knee joints: systematic review and economic evaluation. Health Technol Assess (Winchester, England). 2005;9(47):iii–iv. ix–x, 1–82.

97. Samuelson EM, Brown DE. Cost-effectiveness analysis of autologous chondrocyte implantation: a comparison of periosteal patch versus type I/III collagen membrane. Am J Sports Med. 2012;40(6):1252–8.

98. Minas T. Chondrocyte implantation in the repair of chondral lesions of the knee: economics and quality of life. Am J Orthop (Belle Mead, NJ). 1998;27(11):739–44.

99. Frappier J, Stanish W, Brittberg M, Steinwachs M, Crowe L, Castelo D, et al. Economic evaluation of BST-CarGel as an adjunct to microfracture vs microfracture alone in knee cartilage surgery. J Med Econ. 2014;17(4):266–78.

Periarticular Knee Osteotomy

6

Fernando Corbi, Rosa Ballis, Nicolas Gaggero, and Sebastien Lustig

Contents

F. Corbi, MD • R. Ballis, MD • N. Gaggero, MD
Department of Orthopaedic Surgery,
Hôpital de la Croix-Rousse, Centre Albert Trillat,
103 Grande Rue de La Croix Rousse,
Lyon 69004, France

S. Lustig, MD, PhD (✉)
Department of Orthopaedic Surgery,
Hôpital de la Croix-Rousse, Centre Albert Trillat,
103 Grande Rue de La Croix Rousse,
Lyon 69004, France

Albert Trillat Center, Lyon North University Hospital,
103 Grande Rue de La Croix Rousse,
Lyon 69004, France
e-mail: sebastien.lustig@gmail.com

6.1 High Tibial Osteotomy

6.1.1 Introduction

In valgus and varus knee malalignment in relatively young and active patients, osteotomy has long been recognized as an appropriate option in the management of knee osteoarthritis. Historically, the first high tibial osteotomy (HTO) was performed by Jackson in 1958 with a ball and socket osteotomy below the anterior tibial tuberosity and osteotomy at the middle third of the fibula [1]. Gariepy performed the osteotomy above the anterior tibial tubercle and reported good results in patients with knee osteoarthritis. Following these experiences, HTO was used by several authors. In the same period, opening wedge technique of HTO was developed in France [3, 4] with medial approach, using allograft or autograft bone and plates that allowed stable fixation. At the end of the 1970s, another technique was described by Maquet: the tibial

© ISAKOS 2016
D.A. Parker (ed.), *Management of Knee Osteoarthritis in the Younger, Active Patient:*
An Evidence-Based Practical Guide for Clinicians, DOI 10.1007/978-3-662-48530-9_6

dome osteotomy [5]. After years of popularity, between the 1960s and 1980s, HTO had a slow decline after good results were demonstrated with unicondylar and total knee arthroplasty and rising surgeon preferences for these techniques.

Currently HTO is undergoing a revival, particularly in younger more active patients, due to the desire to preserve the native knee, bone stock, and proprioception and also the possibility to allow physical activities that are not well tolerated with a unicompartmental knee arthroplasty (UKA) [6]. The preference also relates to expectations for physical activities due to the increase in life expectancy [7]. In addition, HTO has become a better option due to new hardware: plates that work like an "internal fixation" allowing a very stable osteosynthesis and periosteal vascular supply preservation. There are also new and more sophisticated bone substitutes and biomaterials that can avoid an iliac crest bone graft harvest and therefore an additional incision with related complications [3, 8, 9].

The first aim of HTO is to eliminate or reduce pain, translating loads to the contralateral femorotibial compartment by correcting deformity. Surgical indications and careful preoperative planning are important to permit long-term satisfying results [10–17]. This chapter will summarize the current knowledge about periarticular knee osteotomies.

6.1.2 Indications and Contraindications (Table 6.1)

Physical indications include: age between 30 and 70 years; well localized pain at the femorotibial joint line; flexion more than 90° and, if present, a lack of extension <10°; normal or correctable ligamentous status (but anterior cruciate ligament [ACL] or posterior cruciate ligament [PCL] insufficiency is not a contraindication); non-reducible deformity; and patients with an active lifestyle [18].

Physical contraindications include obesity, inflammatory disease, smoking, osteoarthritis or meniscectomy in the contralateral compartment, and tibial subluxation more than 1 cm.

Radiological indications include partial or complete joint space width narrowing in one compartment, no contralateral femorotibial joint space width narrowing or patellofemoral joint space width narrowing, and extra-articular deformity more than 5° [18]. MRI can also be used to more accurately assess the contralateral compartment.

Disputable contraindications include patellofemoral arthritis, flexion less than 100° or fixed flexion deformity, severe extra-articular deformity, older than 70 years, and obese female [18] (Table 6.1).

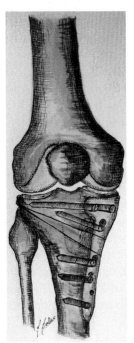

Fig. 6.1 HTO – medial opening wedge

Table 6.1 Indications and contraindications in HTO

Indications	Contraindications
Age between 40 and 70	BMI >30 (disputable)
Flexion >90°, lack of extension <20°	Flexion <90°, lack of extension >20°
Medial femorotibial compartment involvement	Osteoarthritis (3–4° Outerbridge) in contralateral compartment
Non-reducible deformity	Medial meniscectomy
Metaphyseal varus	Infection
Active lifestyle	Rheumatoid arthritis
Good compliance for rehabilitation	Tibial subluxation >1 cm
	High smokers

6.1.3 Surgical Techniques

Two techniques have been used for the treatment of medial compartment arthritis: medial opening wedge high tibial osteotomy (OWHTO) (Fig. 6.1) and lateral closing wedge high tibial osteotomy (CWHTO) (Fig. 6.2).

6.1.3.1 Surgical Planning (Table 6.2)

Preoperatively, a complete radiological evaluation of the limb is mandatory for accurate planning. This is to determine the mechanical axis and calculate the amount of correction required. The standard x-ray series shows the osteoarthritis grade and the tibial slope, including x-rays done in Rosenberg view (45° of flexion). The weight-bearing anteroposterior long-leg x-ray allows measurement of the HKA angle to plan the correction. The axial patellar x-ray assesses involvement of the femoropatellar joint. A guide to the measurement of the constitutional varus is the epiphyseal axis as defined by Levigne (a line connecting the middle of the tibial joint line and the middle of the line connecting the tibial epiphysis). This axis forms a constant angle of $90° \pm 2°$ to the lateral tibial plateau. The constitutional deformity of the tibia is defined as the angle between the epiphyseal and the tibial mechanical axis. The alignment goal of correction for osteoarthritis is usually 2–3° of mechanical valgus [18].

6.1.3.2 Opening Wedge High Tibial Osteotomy (Table 6.3)

The osteotomy is performed just proximal to the tibial tubercle, having elevated the superficial medial collateral ligament. The plane of the osteotomy is horizontal, slightly different from the medial closing wedge HTO, which is more oblique. First two Kirschner wires are introduced medially. Laterally, these guide pins should be just superior to the head of the fibula. Correct position of the guide pins is assessed using the image intensifier. The direction can be adjusted, if necessary. Using an oscillating saw, the tibial cut is made underneath these guide pins, always staying in contact with them. Firstly, the center of the tibia is cut, followed by the anterior and posterior cortices. The cuts are completed using an osteotome, especially on the anterior cortex, where the patellar tendon is at risk. It is necessary to have an intact lateral hinge for this type of osteotomy. Subsequently, a Lambotte osteotome is introduced into the osteotomy. A second osteotome is then introduced below the first. To open up the osteotomy gently, several more osteotomes are introduced between the first two. In order to maintain the tibial slope, the opening of the osteotomy at the posteromedial cortex should

Table 6.2 X-ray needed for a correct planning

Preoperative planning
Standard x-ray posteroanterior and lateral
X-ray in Rosenberg view
Weight-bearing anteroposterior long-leg x-ray
Sky view patellar x-ray

Table 6.3 HTO techniques

Approach and technical considerations
Lateral closing wedge high tibial osteotomy (using a blade plate)
Slightly oblique anterolateral skin incision, the insertion of the tibialis anterior is released as a Z-plasty; tibialis anterior and long toe extensor muscle are released from the metaphysis
Osteotomy of the fibular neck, protect the peroneal nerve
HTO is done proximal to the tibial tubercle in an oblique direction, using image intensifier
Introduce the blade plate, perform the distal cut of the osteotomy with the saw; the medial cortex is weakened with a 3.2 mm drill
Evaluate the femorotibial axis and fix the osteotomy with two bicortical screws
Medial opening wedge high tibial osteotomy
Anteromedial skin incision just proximal to the tibial tubercle, retraction of pes anserinus tendons, incision of the superficial MCL
Perform the osteotomy proximal to the tibial tubercle, first insert two Kirschner guide pins, from medial to lateral, just above the fibular head, use image intensifier; if the position is okay, perform the osteotomy with the saw; first cut the center then the anterior and finally the posterior part of the tibia. Complete the cuts with osteotome
Subsequently introduce a Lambotte osteotome to open the osteotomy and then introduce as much osteotomes as necessary to obtain the desired correction
Fix the osteotomy with a plate and screws or staples

Fig. 6.2 HTO – lateral closing wedge

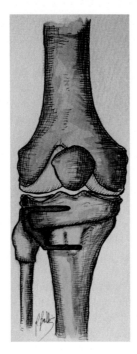

be approximately twice that at the tibial tubercle [19].

Due to autograft site harvest morbidity, bone substitutes have been used with more frequency, mostly of calcium and phosphate. These substitutes try to reproduce the bone structure, with their porosity, provide a structural support, and allow new vessel and osteoprogenitor cell infiltration promoting new bone formation.

Best results are seen with biomaterials like tricalcium phosphate, calcium phosphate, hydroxyapatite-tricalcium phosphate, and hydroxyapatite only. Substitutes like bioglass, coralline wedges, and combined fillers give high rate of delayed union and nonunion [8].

First treatment with HTO was performed without fixation, but this leads to a high rate of complications including loss of correction, joint stiffness, and patellar tendon contracture. The best fixation is still controversial. Options for fixation include staples, external fixators (axial and circular), and plates (conventional, blade plates, locking plates and with or without spacers). Specific plates such as Puddu plate and

Tomofix have demonstrated a high rate of union and less complications [8].

6.1.3.3 Closing Wedge High Tibial Osteotomy (Table 6.3)

The fibular styloid process is first identified, and this procedure usually starts with the osteotomy of fibular head (or neck) or the release of the proximal tibiofibular joint in order to prevent any impingement with the fibula and to allow a final good correction. The surgeon can measure 60 mm distally from the fibular styloid process, in order to define the zone where the fibular osteotomy should be performed. The area between 68 and 153 mm should be avoided, to prevent peroneal nerve palsy [7].

Once the fibular osteotomy is performed, the distal cut of the closing wedge osteotomy is performed. Many surgeons use a guide pin for the distal cut of the osteotomy. The posterior surface of the tibia is protected by a large periosteal elevator, and the patellar tendon is retracted anteriorly. An oscillating saw is used to make the distal cut. An angled cutting guide (6.8 or 10°) is introduced in the distal cut of the osteotomy, and the proximal cut is then made using this angle. The cutting guide should be introduced and impacted on the medial cortex. An oscillating saw is used. The bone wedge is removed. The medial cortex is weakened with a 3.2 mm drill. The wedge is closed, and using a long metal bar positioned on the center of the femur head and in the middle of the ankle joint, the mechanical femorotibial axis is evaluated. The metal bar should pass just laterally to the lateral tibial spine. Computer-assisted surgery can also be used if available.

The osteotomy can be fixed with staples, blade plate, or locking plates.

6.1.4 Results (Tables 6.4 and 6.5)

6.1.4.1 Outcomes

There are 25 published series of high tibial osteotomy with an average of more than 10 years of follow-up currently in the literature [3, 6, 7, 9–12, 16, 20–35]. The studies were divided into two groups: opening wedge high tibial osteotomy

Table 6.4 Systematic review HTO (closing wedge)

Author	Journal/year	Average age	Osteoarthritis classification	Cohort (operated knees)	Device used	Follow-up (years)	Preop average angle	Postop average angle	Results	Scores	Compli-cation rates	Compli-cations	Survival
Gstöttner et al. [6]	Arch Orthop Trauma (2008)	54 years (19–74)	–	134	Staple	12.4 years (1–25)	FTA varus 6–10° 57 %, 11–15° 21 %, 1–5° 18 %	FTA valgus (1 year fu) 1–5° 60 %, 0–5° 20 %, 5–10° 20 %	Survivorship: 94 % 5 years fu, 80 % 10 years fu, 65.5 % 15 years fu, 54 % 18 years fu; predictor factors: age. Not predictor factors: gender, mechanical axis	–	28 %	7 % DVT, 5 % peroneal nerve palsy, 2 % sup infection, 14 % delayed union	39 % converted to TKA
Papachristou et al. [7]	International Orthopaedics (2006)	51 years (26–60)	Ahlbäch 32 % grade I, 23% grade II, 45 % grade III	44	Staple	10 years (5–17)	FTA 177.7°	FTA 185.8°	Postop: 88 % pain relief. 10 years fu: 27.2 % excellent, 9.09 % good, 11.3 % fair-poor. 10–15 year fu: 4.5 % excellent, 15.9 % good, 15.8 % fair-poor	HSSK preop: 52 points. HSSK postop: 83.5 points excellent-good, 58.83 points fair-poor	11 %	4.5 % Sup. infection, 4.5 % tibial fracture, 1 % pulmonary embolism	–

(continued)

Table 6.4 (continued)

Author	Journal/year	Average age	Osteoarthritis classification	Cohort (operated knees)	Device used	Follow-up (years)	Preop average angle	Postop average angle	Results	Scores	Complication rates	Complications	Survival
Koshino et al. [8]	The Knee (2006)	59.6 years (40–73)	Ahlbäck 60% grade II, 35% grade III, 6% grade IV	241	Plate + screws	68 knees included 19 years (15–28)	FTA 186°±6.5°	FTA 171°±7.5°	15–28 years fu: 98% satisfied	HSSK preop: 21% 60–69 points ffair.78% 59 points poor. HSSK postop: 65% 85–100 points excellent, 25% 70–84 points good, 10% 60–69 points fair	6%	4.4% peroneal nerve palsy, 1.4% tibial fracture	16% converted to TKA/MUA at final fu
Aoki et al. [32]	JBJS (2006)	59.8 years (47–72)	HUGS 25% grade II, 55% grade III, 20% grade IV	86	External fixator	56 knees included 11 years (10–15)	FTA 185.4° (180–198°)	FTA 170.6° (163–183°)	18% good, 45% fair, 37% poor	TKSS preop: 53.2 (35–65), poor. Postop: 74.4 (50–95), fair	28%	23% delayed union, 3% peroneal nerve palsy, 2% superficial infection	3% converted to TKA
Sprenger et al. [5]	JBJS (2003)	69 years (47–81)	Ahlbäck 57% grade I, 54% grade II, 3% grade III	76	Plate + screws	10.8 years	–	–	Survivorship: 86% 5 years fu, 74% 10 years fu, 56% 15 years fu. Mean patient satisfaction 9.5 years. No differences in: age, gender, weight, Ahlbäck (except grade II vs. III)	HSSK <70 points survivorship: mean 7.4 years	21%	43% nerve palsy, others not reported	34% converted TKA

Aglietti et al. [17]	JKS (2003)	58 years (36–69)	–	120	32 % plaster cylinder cast 68 % screw + cylinder cast	61 knees included in 15 years (10–21)	Average varus angle 4.7°±5°	–	Preop pain: 66 % moderate, 33 % severe. Postop pain: 16 % mild, 21 % moderate, no severe pain reported	HSSK final fu: 46 % excellent, 25 % good, 21 % fair, 8 % poor	9 %	4 % DVT, 1 % fatal PE, 5 % delayed union	25 % converted TKA average time conversion 11 years (7–17)
Benzakour et al. [23]	International Orthopaedics (2010)	55 years (40–72)	Ahlbäch 20 % grade I, 35 % grade II, 37 % grade III, 8 % grade IV	106	Plate/staples/molded cast	15 years (5–27)	Average varus angle 11°	–	12 % excellent, 30 % good, 31 % fair, 27 % poor	HSSK improvement: 86 % score improvement at final fu	11 %	2 % implant removal, 2 % sup infection, 1 % hematoma, 1 % art. fracture, 2 % cortical fracture, 1 % DVT, 1 % nerve palsy, 2 % dystrophy	10 % converted TKA, 2 % re-osteotomy

(continued)

Table 6.4 (continued)

Author	Journal/year	Average age	Osteoarthritis classification	Cohort (operated knees)	Device used	Follow-up (years)	Preop average angle	Postop average angle	Results	Scores	Complication rates	Complications	Survival
Douglas et al. [16]	Clin Orthop Relat Res (1999)	55 years (16–76)	–	94	Staples/external fixator	61 knees included in 14 years (10–22)	–	–	Survivorship estimate of failure: 73 % at 5 years, 51 % at 10 years, 39 % at 15 years, 30 % at 20 years. Risk factors associated: >50 years, prev arthroscopy, <120° flexion arch, high BMI, lat thrust	–	20 %	15 % delayed union, 10 % nonunion, 3 % art. fracture, 16 % sup infection, 2 % deep infection, 2 % instability, 25 % DVT, 3 % perrenial nerve palsy	20 % converted TKA at latest fu
Yasuda et al. [19]	Clin Orthop Relat Res (1992)	60 years (47–72)	Sasaki 18 % stage II, 58 % stage III, 24 % stage IV	86	External fixator	51 knees included in 11 years (10–15)	FTA 185.5° (175–185°)	FTA 6 years fu: 169°±5.4°; 10 years fu: 170°±6.3°	Preop: 7 % fair, 93 % poor. 6 years fu: 63 % good, 25 % fair, 12 % poor. 10 years fu: 18 % good, 45 % fair, 37 % poor	TKSS improvement: 54 % 6 years fu, 49 % 10 years fu. WAS improvement: 2 % 6 years fu, 2 % 10 years fu. PS improvement: 4 % 6 years fu, 3 % 10 years fu	5 %	2 % peroneal nerve palsy, 1 % sup infection, 1 % delayed union	2 % converted TKR <5 years of fu

Study	Journal	Age	Grade	No.	Fixation	Knees/follow-up	Average varus angle	Postop	Outcome		Score	%	Complications	Conversion
Fletcher et al. [22]	Clin Orthop Relat Res (2006)	42 years (15–76)	Ahlbäch 64 % grade I, 28 % grade II, 8 % grade III	372	Staple/ plate + screws	301 knees included in 18 years (12–28)	Average varus angle 6° (13–15°)	66 % postop varus deformity 5° (1–12°)/ 34 % postop valgus deformity 3° (1–10°)	33 % excellent, 44 % good, 7 % fair, 15 % poor protecting factors outcome: <50 year, BMI <25, Ahlbäch grade I, postop valgus angle >6°. No correlation: gender; preop varus angle	–		3 %	1 % DVT, 1 % sympathetic dystrophies, 1 % fixation failure, 0.3 % other complications	7 % converted TKA/4 % converted MUA revision end point 8 years
Majima et al. [18]	Clin Orthop Relat Res (2000)	59 years (47–70)	–	48	External fixator	26 knees included in 12 years (10–15)	FTA 185.1± 6.3°	FTA 171° ±6.1°	–		TKSS preop: 7 % fair, 93 % poor. Postop: 1 year 49 % good, 51 % fair, 1 % poor. 10 years 17 % good, 44 % fair, 39 % poor	4 %	4 % skin necrosis. No serious complications observed	4 % converted TKA <7 years fu
Yasuda et al. [20]	Bulletin HJDOT (1991)	59 years (37–76)	HUGS 14 % grade II, 58 % grade III, 27 % grade IV	86	External fixator	55 knees included in 12 years (10–15)	FTA 186° (175–195°)	FTA 170.6° (10 years fu)	Preop: 11 % fair, 89 % poor. 6 year fu: 62 % good, 23 % fair, 15 % poor. 10 year fu: 25 % good, 36 % fair, 38 % poor		TKSS preop: 60.2 points, poor. Postop: (6/10 years fu) 89.7 points, fair; 81.4 points, fair. WAS preop: 11.2. Postop: (6/10 years fu) 17.3, 14.1. PS preop: 13.5. Postop: (6/10 years fu) 27.4, 23.3	7 %	4 % peroneal nerve palsy, 1.5 % delayed union, 1.5 % sup infection	4 % converted TKA <5 years fu

(continued)

Table 6.4 (continued)

Author	Journal/year	Average age	Osteoarthritis classification	Cohort (operated knees)	Device used	Follow-up (years)	Preop average angle	Postop average angle	Results	Scores	Complication rates	Complications	Survival
Ivarson et al. [21]	JBJS (1999)	73 years (52–87)	–	99	Staple	65 knees included in 11.9 years (11–13)	–	–	Satisfaction: 5.7 years fu; 57 % good/78 % acceptable/11, 9 years fu; 43 % good 60 % acceptable pain at rest: prep 65 %/5.7 years fu: 38 %/ 11.9 years fu: 30 %	LST: 11.9 years fu; 64 ± 21; fair	12 %	9 % sup infection, 2 % DVT, 1 % peroneal nerve palsy	6 % converted TKA and 1 % converted MUA <5.7 years fu
Van Raaij et al. [33]	Acta Orthopaedica (2008)	49 years (24–67)	Ahlbäch 5 % grade 0, 43 % grade I, 44 % grade II, 8 % grade III	100	Staple	12 years (10–16)	FTA 6.5°	–	Regression model, high risk to conversion to TKA: woman, Ahlbäch >2. No risk associated with BMI and preop HKA angle	–	4 %	1 % over-correction (varus HTO), 1 % symptomatic exostosis, 3 % peroneal nerve palsy	25 % converted TKA < average of 6 years. Probability of surviving HTO 75 % at 10 years fu

Author	Journal (year)	Age	KLC/grade	N	Fixation	Knees/FU	FTA preop	FTA postop	Survival/Satisfaction	Score		Complications	Conversion/Notes
Schallberger et al. [27]	Knee Surg Sports Traumatol Arthrosc (2011)	40 years (15–68)	–	71	OWHTO: plate+screws. Iliac crest CWHTO: plate+screws	54 knees included in 13.5 years (13–21)	FTA 178° (171–184°)	FTA 190° (184–190°) median correction 10°	Osteotomy survival was of 98% after 5 years, 92% after 10 years, and 71% after 15 years	Average VAS at final fu: 0, range 0–4 (0–10). MSI: 80%, range 30–100 (0–100) at final fu. Median KOOS score: 71, range 9–100. Median WOMAC score: 84, range 9–100, both at final fu	–	–	24% converted TKA, 76% survivor HTO at final fu OWHTO vs. CWHTO no significant difference in survival and score outcome
Babis et al. [29]	J Orthop Sci (2008)	53 years (19–71)	–	54	Plate + screws	36 knees included in 10 years (7–14)	FTA 186.6°±3°	FTA 177.2±3.61 (2 months fu)	Satisfaction 35% excellent, 16% good, 11% fair, 19% poor result or had failed. No risk factors: age, BMI, preop medial load, preop/postop medial line obliquity	HSSK preop: 49 points, poor. At final fu: 77 points, good	–	–	31% converted to TKA <7.6 years fu osteotomy survival rate 89% at 5 years/76% at 10 years
Omori et al. [30]	J Orthop Sci (2008)	59 years (40–69)	KLC 16% grade II, 73% grade III, 10% grade IV	68	Plate + screws	48 knees included in 17.1 years (14–24)	FTA 185.4±4.4	FTA 169.1±4.5 (6.5 years fu)/169.8±5.2 (17.1 years fu)	77% satisfied, 33% unsatisfied	JOA score 48 knees. Preop: 59.1 points, poor. 6.5 years fu: 86.3 points, good. >10 years fu: 83.1 points, good	4%	2% peroneal nerve palsy, 2% delayed union	–

(continued)

Table 6.4 (continued)

Author	Journal/year	Average age	Osteoarthritis classification	Cohort (operated knees)	Device used	Follow-up (years)	Preop average angle	Postop average angle	Results	Scores	Compli-cation rates	Compli-cations	Survival
Akizuki et al. [28]	JBJS (2008)	63 years (45–76)	KLC 6 % grade II, 33 % grade III, 61 % grade IV	132	Plate + screws	94 knees included in 16.4 years (16–20)	FTA 183.7° (177–195)	–	74 % excellent/good at final fu	HSSK preop: 60.7 points, fair. 5 years fu: 90 points, excellent. Final fu: 84 points. Good risk factors: BMI, prep range of movement	13 %	4.2 % peroneal nerve palsy, 0.8 % DVT, 2.5 % skin necrosis, 0.8 % sup infection, 1.6 % nonunion, 1.6 % early loss correction	7.4 % converted to TKA. Survivorship 97.6 % at 10 years fu/90.4 % at 15 years fu
Hoells et al. [31]	JBJS (2014)	50 years (26–66)	1 % mild, 10 % moderate, 89 % severe	164	Plate + screws	95 knees included in 10 years	–	–	Improved survival rates: age <50 year, BMI <30, WOMAC >45	WOMAC: preop. 61/5 years fu; 88 /10 years fu: 84 TKSS: prep 130/5 years fu; 181/10 years fu; 168	7 %	1 % PE, 2 % sup infection. 3 % delayed union, 1 % nonunion	Survivorship 87 % at 5 years of fu/79 % at 10 years fu

Fu follow-up

Table 6.5 High tibial osteotomy (opening wedge)

Author	Journal/year	Average age	Side	Osteoarthritis classification	Cohort (operated knees)	Device used	Graft	Follow-up (years)	Preop average angle	Postop average angle	Results	Scores	Complication rates	Complications	Survival
Hernigou et al. [13]	The knee (2001)	59 years (35–73)	Medial opening wedge	–	245	Plate + screws	Cement block	87 knees included in 10 years (6–15)	–	75 % desired correction (3–6° valgus), 5 % over-corrected, 20 % under-corrected	Survivorship (Kaplan-Meier): 94 % (5 years), 85 % (10 years), 68 % (15 years)	–	4 %	1.6 % postoperative infection, 0.4 % vascular injury, 0.4 % DVT, 0.4 % non-union, 0.8 % delayed union	87 patients (10 years fu): 26.4 % converted TKR, 73.5 % satisfied
Hernigou et al. [11]	International Orthopaedics (2010)	60 years (43–67)	Medial opening wedge	–	53	Plate + screws	Resorbable tricalcium phosphate	10 years (8–12)	FTA 162° (158–165°)	FTA 180° (173–190°) 10–12 years	10 years fu: 81 % excellent-good/1.3 % fair/ 11.3 % poor	–	4 %	3.7 % fixation system complain (before 4 years after OWTO)	9.4 % converted TKA, 1.8 % converted MUA (before 7 years after OWTO)
Marti et al. [14]	JBJS (2001)	43 years (17–66)	Lateral opening wedge	Ahlbäck 41 % grade I, 53 % grade II, 5.8 % grade III	36	Plate 53 % Screw 8.8 % Ext. fix. 3 % Staple 5.8 % None 30 %	Iliac crest	11 years (5–21)	FTA 11.6° (4–22)	FTA 5.1° (–5–13)	0 % progression OA, 0 % loss ROM after follow up	LGS 26 % excellent 62 % good 9 % fair 3 % poor	15 %	9 % nerve palsy, 3 % superficial infection, 3 % thrombo-phlebitis	3 % converted to arthrodesis because severe pain (before 6 years after OWTO)
Benzakour et al. [23]	International Orthopaedics (2010)	55 years (40–72)	Medial opening wedge	Ahlbäck 20 % grade I, 35 % grade II, 37 % grade III, 8 % grade IV	118	Plate/ staples/ molded cast	Iliac crest	15 years (5–27)	FTA 133°	–	12 % excellent/ good/31 % fair/27 % poor	KSS improvement: 67 % score improvement at final fu	11 %	2 % re-osteotomy, 2 % implant removal, 2 % sup. infection, 1 % hematoma, 1 % art. fracture, 2 % cortical fracture, 1 % DVT, 1 % nerve palsy, 2 % dystrophy	10 % converted TKA

(continued)

Table 6.5 (continued)

Author	Journal/year	Average age	Side	Osteoarthritis classification	Cohort (operated knees)	Device used	Graft	Follow-up (years)	Preop average angle	Postop average angle	Results	Scores	Complication rates	Complications	Survival
Hernigou et al. [10]	JBJS (1987)	60 years (43–77)	Medial opening wedge	Ahlbäch 37 % grade I, 48 % grade II, 11 % grade III, 2 % grade IV, 1 % grade V	89	Plate + screws	Iliac crest	76 knees included in 11.5 years (10–30)	FTA 172° (158–179)	FTA 182° (173–190°)	Final follow up preop pain: 55 % severe/49 % moderate/ 5 % mild postop pain: 13 % severe/16 % moderate/ 16 % mild/55 % none	–	–	–	18 % knees required revision at 5–10 years: 5 % MUA, 4 % bicompart-mental,10%re-osteotomy
Saragaglia et al. [15]	International Orthopaedics (2011)	53 years (32–74)	Medial opening wedge	Ahlbäch 22 % grade I, 34 % grade II, 35 % grade III, 9 % grade IV	124	Plate + screws	Tricalcium phosphate	107 knees included in 10 years (8–14)	FTA 172° (162–179°)	FTA 182° (178–186°)	HTO survivorship: 89 % in 5 years/74 % in 10 years 88 % satisfaction at final fu	LS: preop 65.4±13.3 points/postop 88±12.7 points (51–100) KOOS score 86±4.6 points (25–100)	22 %	8 % tibial plateau fracture, 2 % DVT, 3 % PE, 6 % delayed union, 3 % screw breakages	12 % converted TKA at 8±3 years

(OWHTO) and closing wedge high tibial osteotomy (CWHTO).

CWHTO

The CWHTO results included 2091 operated knees. The mean follow-up range is from 10 to 18 years. There are different kinds of devices that have been used to fix the osteotomy: plate and screws 42 %, staples 31 %, external fixture 26 %, and cylinder plaster 1 %. In literature, the average femorotibial angle pre- and post-operation is 177°–186° and 169°–190°, respectively.

Good results have been reported regarding survival rates, >survivorship at 5 years of follow-up from 73 to 98 %, at 10 years of follow-up from 51 to 92 %, and more than 15 years of follow-up from 39 to 71 % [7, 20, 25]. Koshino et al. reported a satisfaction rate at final follow-up for excellent/good results of 98 % at 15–28 years of follow-up [22]. Sprenger et al. reported excellent/good patient satisfaction of 9.5 years after HTO [7].

Risk factors that have been associated with poor outcomes are age more than 50 years at time of surgery, less than 120° of flexion, high BMI, lateral thrust, more than Ahlbäck grade I articular degeneration in contralateral compartment, and excess postoperative valgus angle [10, 22, 25, 30, 31, 35].

Survival rates are influenced by preoperative mechanical axis, gender, and WOMAC >45 [7, 10, 20, 31, 33, 35]. Van Raaij et al. associated low grades of survival rates in women [35]. Conversion rates included for conversion to total knee arthroplasty or unicompartmental arthroplasty are from 3 to 39 % [2, 6, 7, 10, 20, 25, 27–29, 31, 35].

OWHTO

The OWHTO results included 665 operated knees. Literature shows the prevalence of the medial opening osteotomy technique except Marti et al. who perform a lateral opening osteotomy [26]. Mean follow-up range is from 10 to 15 years.

The fixation devices used were plate and screws, staples, screws, external fixator, and modulated cast. Tricortical iliac crest was used in 50 % of the articles, tricalcium phosphate was used in 33 % of the studies, and 16 % used cement block. Average femorotibial angle pre- and post-operation is 133°–172° and 180°–182°, respectively.

Good results have been reported regarding survival rates, survivorship at 5 years of follow-up

from 89 to 94 %, at 10 years of follow-up from 74 to 85 %, and more than 15 years of follow-up around 68 %, reported by Hernigou et al. [9, 24]. Hernigou et al. mentioned a satisfaction rate at 10 years follow-up for excellent/good results of 81 % and Saragaglia et al. 88 % excellent/good results at final follow-up [9, 22].

At 10 years, conversion rates included for conversion to total knee arthroplasty are 10–26 % with 73 % excellent/good satisfaction at the final follow-up [9, 11, 23, 24]. Conversion to unicompartmental arthroplasty ranges from 2 to 35 % [3, 23].

6.1.4.2 Complications (Tables 6.4, 6.5, 6.6 and 6.7)

For CWHTO complication rates, the average is from 3.3 to 28 %. The most frequent complication reported in this group is peroneal nerve palsy with rates from 2 to 43 % [7, 20, 22, 26, 34], followed by delayed union with an average of 2–23 % [6, 20, 25,

Table 6.6 Advantages and disadvantages of the two different techniques

Surgical techniques: advantages and disadvantages
Closing wedge high tibial osteotomy
Lateral
Peroneal nerve palsy
Potentially less accurate
Potential changes in patellar height (patella alta)
Opening wedge high tibial osteotomy
Medial
Fracture of the lateral hinge or the tibial plateau
Creates less deformity than CW in tibial metadiaphysis
Potential increase in tibial posterior tibial slope
Potential changes in patellar height (patella infera)

Table 6.7 Complications in HTO

Complications
Malunion
Nonunion
Patella infera or patella alta
Stiffness
Loss of correction
Hardware failure
Compartment syndrome
Neurologic injury (peroneal nerve palsy)
Vascular injury
Infection
Proximal tibial fracture

32, 34]. Other important complications are deep vein thrombosis, pulmonary embolism, superficial infection, skin necrosis, and sympathetic dystrophies. OWHTO complication rates are 3 to 22 %, mainly due to tibial plateau fracture in 10 %, nerve palsy in 10 %, and delayed union in 10 %. Other important complications are superficial infection and vascular problems [3, 9, 11, 16, 23, 25].

6.1.5   Discussion

Knee joint realignment is intended to redistribute knee joint forces from the affected area to the unaffected side to interrupt the vicious cycle of destruction and malalignment described by Coventry who postulated arbitrarily that varus knees should be overcorrected by osteotomy to 5° of valgus [31]. The majority of authors have reported satisfactory results in the short to midterm, but these results gradually deteriorated over time, especially at more than 10 years after surgery. The most important finding of this review is the high survival rate of HTO which after 5 years of follow-up is over 95 %, after 10 years of follow-up is around 80 %, and more than 15 years of follow-up is more than 50 % for both techniques.

The percentage of satisfactory results (excellent/good) after HTO was over 80 % after long-term follow-up for both techniques. Looking at patients converted to TKA, most operations were performed more than 10 years after HTO. Generally, osteoarthritis progressed, and increasing symptoms became the indication for further surgery. Total knee arthroplasty should be reserved for unicompartmental or bicompartmental diseases in older and/or lower demand patients [29]. The success of osteotomies depends primarily on correct indication. Patients should have good pain tolerance because a low pain threshold is often a negative factor in the outcome of the treatment of musculoskeletal disease. Precise planning and appropriate surgical technique achieving the desired correction are fundamental [29]. Aglietti et al. reported that opening wedge technique creates less deformity than the closing with tibial metadiaphyseal mismatch that might interfere with a subsequent revision to TKA [6]. But hinge position can affect the change in posterior tibial slope. Medial OWHTO, in particular, is associated with an increased posterior slope (PTS) compared to CWHTO, due to an increased anterior positioning of the wedge. Anterior and superior translation of tibial plateau is followed by an earlier contact with femoral condyle. CWHTO is more commonly associated with a decrease in PTS. El-Azab et al. described PTS in OWHTO preop/postop with locking and no locking plate, 7.7°/9.1° and 5°/8.1°, respectively, and PTS in CWHTO preop/postop of 5.7°/2.4° [36]. Understanding of anatomy, and careful surgical technique can avoid unintentional changes in tibial slope.

Regarding the patellar height CWHTO is associated with an increased patellar height due to lowering the joint line, and in OWHTO descent of the patella is constant. Tigiani et al. observed a patella elevation in 57 % of CWHTO (Caton-Deschamps index), associated with a postoperation correction of knee axis less than 10°. OWHTO postoperation knee axis correction more than 15° is associated with a patella baja [37].

Regarding the filler used Lash et al. detailed that allograft is used in 25.9 %, autograft 29.5 %, tricalcium phosphate 12.6 %, calcium phosphate 7.2 %, hydroxyapatite-tricalcium phosphate 3.4 % (which is associated with higher rates of loss of correction), bioglass 1.7 %, combined fillers 0.9 %, coralline wedge 0.9 %, hydroxyapatite 0.4 %, and no filler 17.3 % [8].

For Benzakour et al. opening technique did not give significantly better clinical outcome than closing technique [11]. Opening and closing wedge HTO have similar results in functional outcome and survival. Literature comparing clinical outcome after opening versus closing wedge HTO is very limited and long-term comparisons are lacking, with only two authors reporting the comparison [11, 29]. Our results not only confirm the long-term effectiveness of valgisation high tibial osteotomy as treatment for medial compartment osteoarthritis, but there is also evidence that the opening wedge technique can have a long-lasting effect similar to the traditional closing wedge high tibial osteotomy. This has a high clinical relevance currently, as an increasing percentage of HTO are done using the opening wedge technique, and long-term experiences are very limited [29]. The main reason for the good clinical outcome is the good alignment which has been described as the most important factor for good long-term clinical results [22].

There is still considerable discussion about which factors affect the long-term outcome of HTO. Two of the most important factors are the correction angle at surgery and the preoperative severity of knee osteoarthritis. Regarding the correction angle, previous studies have reported that the optimum clinical outcomes were associated with a correction of 6–16° valgus, and an undercorrection less than 5° was strongly related to a high failure rate [6, 7, 22].

Douglas et al. showed that preoperative knee flexion of less than 120 was related to significantly lower survival, but Aglietti et al. did not relate failure to either flexion contracture or lack of extension. We found that the preoperative range of movement of <100 was significantly associated with early failure [6, 25].

6.1.6 Conclusions

In summary, opening and closing wedge high tibial osteotomies are successful and durable methods of treatment for unicompartmental degenerative diseases with associated varus in active patients. Survival of both techniques is comparable in most series and is associated with low complication rates, high satisfaction, and high activity levels of the survivors.

6.2 Distal Femoral Osteotomy

6.2.1 Introduction

Historically, the first treatment for genu valgum was osteotomy, but with the advent of TKA and UKA, they have been used less commonly. Today, osteotomy represents a valid option which allows postponing TKA and thereby preserving the native knee.

Degeneration of the tibiofemoral compartment leads to a valgus deformity that is frequently a consequence of partial or total lateral meniscectomy. Other causes are post-traumatic, partial

epiphysiodesis and growth disorders. The purpose of osteotomies around the valgus knee is to relieve the lateral knee compartment and to displace the loads medially.

Proximal tibial varus osteotomy can be used for minor genu valgum deformities, but not for major angulations, or if the projected obliquity of the joint is more than 10°. Distal femoral osteotomy (DFO) is a good option because tibial osteotomies for large deformities produce medial tilt of the joint line, which may increase lateral shear forces and lateral subluxation during gait [5]. The most commonly performed techniques are the lateral opening or the medial closing, with dome osteotomy rarely used [38–40].

The aim of this section is to analyze the literature about DFO regarding indications, results, functional outcomes, and survivorship.

6.2.2 Indications and Contraindications (Table 6.8)

Appropriate indications for DFO are critical for final stability and good outcomes [40, 41]. Painful valgus deformity with related osteoarthritis in the lateral compartment is the absolute indication for

Table 6.8 List of indications and contraindications of DFO

Indications	Contraindications
Age <60 male, age <55 female	BMI >30 (disputable)
Flexion >90°, lack of extension <20°	Flexion <90°, lack of extension >20°
Lateral femorotibial compartment involvement	Osteoarthritis (3–4° Outerbridge) in medial compartment
Mechanical angle deformity localized in the femur	Medial meniscectomy
Genu valgum	Infection
Active lifestyle	Rheumatoid arthritis
Good compliance for rehabilitation	Tibial subluxation >1 cm
	Valgus deformity >20° (disputable)
	High smoking

DFO [42–46]. Better results have been seen in patients with mild osteoarthritis [47] and in valgus deformity not more than 20° due to the significant ligamentous laxity [48]. McDermott et al. stated that arthritis of the medial knee compartment is not an absolute contraindication, as long as it is minor compared to the lateral compartment. In addition, there must be good bone stock, normal circulation, a stable joint, and knee flexion >90° [15]. A small lack of extension may be tolerated and corrected during surgery [49].

Absolute contraindications include severe osteoarthritis of the medial compartment of the knee, severe tricompartmental osteoarthritis, and tibiofemoral subluxation [44, 46]. Osteoporosis is a relative contraindication because, despite a rigid femoral fixation, the cortical bone of the proximal segment can often subside into the cancellous bone of the distal segment when the patient weight-bears, resulting in unwanted axial deviation [45].

For Stahelin et al. contraindications are also valgus deformity due to obliquity of the tibial plateau, inflammatory arthritis, instability due to laxity of the medial collateral ligament, lack of extension >15°, and severe osteoporosis [45]. Puddu et al. included BMI >30 and severe bone loss (more than a few millimeters) of the lateral tibia or femur, since after intervention congruent weight-bearing on both tibial plateaus is not possible [48].

Femoropatellar involvement for Stahelin et al. is an absolute contraindication [45], but Zarrouck et al. and Wang et al. treated, respectively, nine patients and eight patients with DFO associated with patellofemoral osteoarthritis in which they performed a lateral release in 15 patients, distal realignment in one, and combined proximal and distal realignment in one patient. The final results at last follow-up were satisfactory [43, 46]. The proposed reason is because distal varus osteotomy decreases the Q angle between the quadriceps tendon and the patellar tendon, which reduces the magnitude of the patella's lateral traction forces [5].

6.2.3 Surgical Technique (Table 6.9)

Tibial medial closing wedge osteotomy was the first technique performed, but results have been

Table 6.9 DFO surgical techniques

Approach and technical considerations
Medial closing wedge distal femoral osteotomy
Approach medial side, proximal to the adductor tubercle and the anterior side of the femoral articular surface
Osteotomy technique osteotomy trait parallel to the joint line. Do x-ray to ascertain that the chisel has not penetrated the intercondylar notch or the anterior femoral surface. Important to leave untouched the lateral cortex. Removal of a 5–10 mm bone wedge from the distal femur. Fixation with different hardware mostly a 90°degree offset dynamic compression blade plate or Tomofix
Lateral opening wedge distal femoral osteotomy
Approach lateral side, distal third of the femur 15 cm proximal to the joint line until the Gerdy's tubercle, carried down from the vastus lateralis muscle
Osteotomy technique If deformity is metaphyseal, osteotomy cut must be parallel and 30 mm proximal to the joint line; if diaphyseal it must be oblique to the joint line. Opening wedge filled up with auto-allograft, PRP, and bone cement and fixed with different hardware mostly the 95° blade plate, Puddu plate, or Tomofix

reported not to be as good as those of proximal tibial valgus osteotomy for varus deformity. For corrections more than 12° of valgus, HTO is not recommended because the joint line, after bone removal, will be oblique medially inducing an increase in femorotibial shear stress. DFO will give much better results at long follow-up. Actually, the most commonly performed is the medial closing DFO as reported in multiple studies [42, 45, 46, 48–63].

All authors agree with regard to preoperative assessment: standard x-ray posteroanterior and lateral in which the tibial slope can be assessed, AP x-ray in Rosenberg view to quantify the compartmental involvement of osteoarthritis, weight-bearing anteroposterior long-leg x-ray to measure the angle deformity between the femur and tibia (mechanical or anatomic axis) and calculate the desired correction, and axial view of the patella to evaluate any osteoarthritis in the femoropatellar joint (Table 6.8). MRI scan is also a useful supplement to more accurately assess articular cartilage pathology.

6.2.3.1 Technique: Medial Closing Wedge DFO (Fig. 6.3)

With the knee joint in the extended position, an anteromedial longitudinal incision is made starting 10 cm above the patella and ending at the upper third of the patella. This incision has the advantage that it can be used again for any subsequent surgery. Incise the subcutaneous tissue and dissect the fascia of the vastus medialis muscle. Elevate the muscle and dissect as far as necessary from the intermuscular septum. Expose the medial patellofemoral ligament at the distal end of the incision. Incise the ligament and the distal insertion of the vastus medialis muscle in order to facilitate mobilization of the muscle. Now expose the intermuscular septum near the condyles and incise the septum carefully, close to the bone and parallel to the femoral shaft. Separate the soft tissue of the back of the knee from the distal femur, to allow the use of a wide, blunt-tipped Hohmann retractor behind the femoral shaft. Use a Hohmann retractor to expose the anteromedial aspect of the supracondylar region of the femur. Expose the shaft proximally so that the plate can be positioned safely.

The position of the osteotomy is best determined by placing the plate directly on the anteromedial distal femur. It is not necessary to achieve a distal fit due to the angular stability. However, it is important to ensure that the distal screws do not penetrate the condyles dorsally.

The distal osteotomy cut should be placed approximately 5 mm above the patella groove descending laterally, ending 10 mm from the lateral cortical bone in the lateral condyle of the femur (Table 6.10). The proximal osteotomy starts higher in the medial supracondylar region. It is advisable to mark the planned osteotomy site with an electric cautery.

Perform the osteotomies by marking the planned wedge removal with Kirschner wires (check the Kirschner wire placement with the image intensifier before cutting). The wires will then act as a guide for the saw. The osteotomy ends 10 mm before the lateral cortical bone, leaving a lateral hinge and removing a medially based wedge. Perform the osteotomies with an oscillating saw, protecting the soft tissue with a Hohmann retractor and constantly cooling the saw blade. Remove the wedge; check that any residual bone fragments have been removed from the osteotomy. If the bone is very hard, weaken the lateral cortical bone with the 2.5 mm drill bit.

Close the osteotomy carefully by applying continuous pressure to the lateral lower limb while stabilizing the knee joint region. This may take several minutes. The osteotomy gap can then either be held closed by manual compression or with two crossed Kirschner wires considering the later plate position. Check the corrected mechanical axis with the image intensifier by positioning a long metal rod between the center of the femoral head and the center of the ankle joint. The projected axis line passes either centrally or just medial to the center of

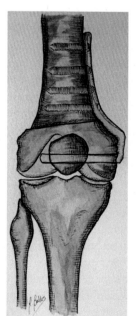

Fig. 6.3 DFO – medial closing wedge

Table 6.10 X-ray pool for preoperative planning

Preoperative planning
Standard x-ray posteroanterior and lateral
X-ray in Rosenberg view
Weight-bearing anteroposterior long-leg x-ray
Sky view patellar x-ray

the knee joint, depending on the preoperative plan.

Position the plate anteromedially on the distal femur. The screws should be aimed in a slightly proximal, lateral direction to achieve good interfragmentary compression. This is particularly important if the lateral femoral cortical bone fractures when closing the osteotomy. Close the arthrotomy and reattach the medial patellofemoral ligament and the partially released distal insertion of the vastus medialis muscle on the patella. Close the wound layer by layer. Although nonunion is uncommon with good surgical technique, even using a locking plate cannot completely eliminate bone healing complications [53].

6.2.3.2 Lateral Opening Wedge Distal Femoral Osteotomy (Using Blade Plate) (Fig. 6.4)

With the knee in 90° of flexion, a lateral skin incision starts 15 cm proximal to the joint line and ends at the level of Gerdy's tubercle. The fascia lata is incised slightly anteriorly in the direction of its fibers, and the lateral vastus muscle is elevated. The perforating arteries of the vastus late-

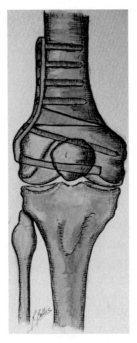

Fig. 6.4 DFO – lateral opening wedge

ralis are carefully coagulated or ligated. Subsequently, the vastus lateralis is elevated from the lateral border of the femoral diaphysis using a periosteal elevator. The patellar tendon is identified and a limited lateral arthrotomy is performed; this exposes the orientation of the trochlea and condyles. Two guide pins are inserted into the joint, one at the femorotibial joint line and the other in the patellofemoral joint. The guide pins help guide the blade plate and reduce the radiation caused by image intensifier.

The osteotomy is horizontal, just proximal to the lateral part of the trochlea. With the knee in extension, the suprapatellar pouch is elevated, and, with the knee at 90° of flexion, the posterior side of the metaphyseal region is elevated. A landmark is made on the lateral side of the femur with the oscillating saw, perpendicular to the horizontal osteotomy. This will serve as a guide to determine the rotation.

The blade should be introduced into the epiphyseal region, 30 mm proximal to the joint line. The blade plate is 5.6 mm thick and 16 mm wide, and the distance between the screw holes is 16 mm. The guide for the blade plate should be introduced ventrally and proximally to the femoral insertion of the lateral collateral ligament. The angle of insertion depends on the level of the deformation. If the deformation is located at the diaphyseal level, the blade should be introduced oblique to the joint line. To obtain a varisation of 10°, the angle should be set at 75° (85–10°) at a complementary angle to the anatomic distal femoral angle (95°, angle of correction). If the deformation is situated at the metaphyseal level, the blade should be introduced parallel to the joint line (this is the most common situation). When introducing the blade parallel to the joint line, a correction to a normal anatomic femoral valgus of 5° is automatically obtained by introducing a 95° angled blade plate. In other words, if the femur were normal, no correction would be obtained if the blade plate is introduced parallel to the joint line. If we are confronted with a combined deformation or with a mixed metaphyseal component (lateral condyle hypoplasia or diaphyseal malunion), the angle of introduction should be even smaller, and the blade plate should be introduced at a smaller angle. Preoperative planning is essential to evaluate the correction needed.

The position of the blade can be checked using the image intensifier. The angle of correction can now be measured on a printout by drawing a line tangent to the medial and lateral condyles and another line tangent to the blade. The femoral osteotomy is performed with an oscillating saw. The medial cortex should not be cut. Once the blade plate is introduced, the medial cortex is fragmented using a drill bit. Two or more osteotomes are then introduced into the osteotomy, but it is the impaction of the blade plate that will progressively open up the osteotomy once in contact with the diaphysis. A screw is temporarily placed in the distal oval screw hole, in the proximal zone of the hole.

The blade plate is now impacted. Subsequently, a screw is introduced into another screw hole while the former screw is taken out. The impaction of the blade plate is continued, and the osteotomy will progressively open up until the blade plate is in full contact with the lateral side of the femoral diaphysis. Progressive impaction allows opening of the osteotomy. Provisional fixation with one screw helps control the correction and provides additional stability. By playing with the impaction and positioning of the screws, one can increase or decrease the amount of opening. If the blade plate is impacted with the screw left in place, the correction will be halted. Conversely, if an additional screw is again placed in the distal part of the screw hole and the former screw is taken out, the correction can be increased.

Final fixation of the blade plate is achieved by four 4.5 mm cortical screws. In lateral opening DFO it is important to graft the osteotomy gap. Different authors have suggested using bone filler for defects greater than 7.5 mm [47], while the gold standard is represented by tricortical iliac crest bone graft. There are different ways to fill the defect as seen in literature with no major complications and substantially good results: allograft, synthetic bone substitutes (hydroxyapatite, β-tricalcium phosphate, bone cement) filled with or without PRP, and growth factors or bone marrow stem cells [13]. Some authors did not use

any graft [42]. The soft tissues and skins are closed over a drain, which is introduced underneath the fascia lata.

6.2.3.3 Hardware Selection

Hardware choice may have an important role because it allows stability of the osteotomy and reliable healing. Blade plate is the hardware mostly utilized and usually demonstrates good results in DFO at long-term follow-up and in the immediate postoperative period and early rehabilitation. For lateral opening osteotomy, plate with less volume leads to better results in terms of iliotibial tract irritation [72].

Edgerton et al. tried different ways of fixation with staples but with poor results and high complication rates. In the recent times, healing will occur reliably also with angle-stabilized locking plate [52]. Van Heerwaarden et al. performed an incomplete medial closing osteotomy with lateral cortical intact to improve final stability of the construct [49].

6.2.3.4 Angle Correction

This remains controversial, and the majority of authors recommend correction of the mechanical axis to $0° + -2$ – the amount of the neutral tibio-femoral angle [14, 16, 42, 46, 48, 49, 51–53, 55, 57–64, 67, 69, 73]. In the average person, the hip-knee-shaft angle is between 5°and 7°. The mechanical axis, on the other hand, is 90° to the same condylar line. Thus, if the anatomic angle is brought to an angle of 90° with the condylar line, the leg will be moved out to the natural valgus approximately 5–7°, and the lateral compartment will be unloaded [59, 73].

McDermott et al. and Cameron et al. found no correlation between alignment and outcome and both aim for an angle of correction of 0° [16, 42]. Some authors, on the basis of Maquet indications, recommend a femoral supracondylar osteotomy with slight overcorrection (in varus) with the object of diminishing considerably the pressure on the joint and distributing the loads uniformly and neutralize the force of medial muscles [6, 47, 50, 54].

Some authors recommend undercorrection retaining a 2–4° of valgus [43, 45, 56, 66]. Some authors did the correction of the mechanical axis to a line passing the knee joint just medial to the deepest point of the trochlea [49, 61, 74].

Marin Morales et al. found, in line with the study of Sharma et al. [75] about the role of knee alignment in OA disease progression and functional decline, that malalignment greater than 5° (varus or valgus) was associated with a significantly greater functional deterioration over the period of follow-up.

6.2.4 Results (Tables 6.11, 6.12, 6.13, and 6.14)

6.2.4.1 Outcomes

Medial femoral closing wedge is the most commonly used technique for the correction of valgus alignment, since McDermott et al. described this technique. They removed a wedge between 5 and 10 mm, showing good results in 92 % of 24 patients treated with DFO [16]. With a similar technique, Healy et al. reported good results in 86 % of 23 patients, with a mean correction of ±2° of valgus [56].

Learmonth, using a special jig for tibial anatomic axis alignment, achieved good results in 20 osteotomies after a mean of 4 years with no complications [60]. Finkelstein et al. showed good results in 64 % at 11 years follow-up, with complications attributed to poor selection of patients [53].

Wang et al. reported survivorship in 30 osteotomies of 87 % at 10 years follow-up and did not recommend articular debridement associated with DFO as it increased the risk of postoperative arthrofibrosis [46]. Backstein et al. described a DFO survivorship of 82 % at 10 years follow-up and 45 % at 15 years follow-up of 38 knees [6]. Similar results were reported by Gross et al. who found good results at 10 years follow-up with survivorship of about 64 % [62].

Koshashvili et al. reported at 1 year follow-up excellent/good results in 84.4 % of patients. Failure rate at 15.8 years follow-up was about 48.5 % [55]. Sternheim et al. reported results at long follow-ups: 89.9 % survival at 10 years, 78.9 % survival at 15 years, and 21.5 % at 20 years of 45 osteotomies done with blade plate [58].

Edgerton et al., in a study of 24 knees, reported a 71 % rate of satisfactory results after an average duration of follow-up of 8.3 years [52]. Mathews et al., in a study of 21 patients who underwent DFO followed by stabilization with a plaster cast, staples, or a blade plate, reported only a 33 % rate of satisfactory results, but he did report high rate of complications after 1–8 years follow-up [47]. Stahelin et al., using a semitubular AO plate, reported improving HSS score in a mean follow-up of 5 years in 21 osteotomies [45]. Similar results were retrieved by Omidi-Kashani et al. at 1.5 years mean follow-up [57].

Freiling et al. reported good results between 3 months and 4 years follow-up using Tomofix in 60 patients. They had three delayed union/non-union, one deep infection, one superficial infection, one hematoma, and one fracture [61]. Similar results were reported by Petersen et al. [62]. Recently, Forkel et al. evaluated 23 patients after surgery with the Tomofix plate, reporting better results than Edgerton but comparable with the results reported by Freiling. He had no major complications and only reported one complication: a loss of correction with the possible reason being breach of the lateral cortex of the femur. Finally he stated that using a locking plate (Tomofix) cannot eliminate completely the bone healing complications [54].

There is less literature available for *lateral opening wedge osteotomy*. However, good results were reported by Madelaine et al. at mean follow-up of 6.7 years using a 95° blade plate; they also found that the osteotomy has no impact on the final leg length [64]. Similar results were reported by Dewilde et al. with a survivorship of 82 % at 7 years follow-up, using bioresorbable calcium phosphate cement to fill the defect [65]. Thein et al. also reported good results in six patients at 6.5 years mean follow-up using tricortical iliac crest bone graft [66]. Das et al., in 16 patients at 3 years follow-up, had the same results using bone allograft to fill the osteotomy gap [67]. Saithna et al. reported a survivorship of 79 % at 5 years follow-up [68]. All authors performed surgery as described by Puddu et al. with a Puddu

Table 6.11 Complications of DFO

Complications (from the most frequent)
Malunion
Nonunion
Stiffness
Loss of correction
Hardware failure
Iliotibial band pain (lateral opening DFO)
Neurologic injury
Vascular injury
Infection
Fracture

Table 6.12 Comparison between the two techniques

Surgical techniques: advantages and disadvantages
Closing wedge distal femoral osteotomy
Medial historically the most performed; shorter bone healing; well tolerated by the patient, complex surgical technique
Opening wedge distal femoral osteotomy
Lateral easier to perform instead of the medial closing; bone correction precise; iliotibial tract plate irritation; longer bone healing

plate. Zarrouck et al. reported good results in 23 patients at mean follow-up of 4.5 years using a 95° blade plate with no grafting [43].

Jacobi et al. used a Tomofix plate in 16 patients, with a mean follow-up of 3.75 years. They ultimately abandoned the opening DFO because of high grade of postoperative complications, in particular iliotibial band irritation and slow healing of osteotomy; however, postoperative outcomes appeared to be satisfactory [69].

Nicolaides et al. performed surgery with insertion of a coralline wedge in the osteotomy site [70]. Cameron I. et al. divided the patients into two groups: osteoarthritis group and joint preservation group. The survivorship was 74 % in the first group and 92 % in the second one, after a follow-up of 5 years using different devices: locking plate Dynafix in 22 patients, Puddu plates in six, and Tomofix in one patient. He reported only one nonunion in the arthritic group [71].

There are some probable *prognostic factors* related to the success of this osteotomy. Cameron et al. reported results of 46 patients with a mean follow-up of 3.5 years and attempted to identify these prognostic factors but did not find any correlation between patient age, sex, time after the intervention, final femorotibial angle or number of degrees of correction, and the final good outcome. Patients with delayed union did not differ significantly from those who did not have a delayed union [42]. Other authors believe that good results may be reached with a rigid fixation, adequate correction, and less advanced osteoarthritis [47]. Under- or overcorrection may contribute to failure [50], and good results are predictable with a correction between 0° and 6° of anatomic valgus [43].

6.2.4.2 Complications (Table 6.11)

Complications involving the two techniques are not infrequent, and they are represented mostly by delayed union and nonunion, stiffness, and hardware failure that are frequently associated with lateral opening wedge osteotomy. In addition in lateral DFO the majority of patients complained about iliotibial band pain because of plate irritation (21–86 % in the literature) [69, 71]. Lateral opening osteotomies theoretically elongate the peroneal nerve at the level of a tight trajectory around the fibular head, but in the follow-up there were no nerve injuries [67]. This technique is simpler than the closing DFO since the lateral approach avoids risk of neurovascular complications and is easier to do and the correction will be more accurate [64].

Edgerton demonstrated 63 % failure related to staple fixation that is therefore thought to be an inadequate fixation technique for femoral osteotomies [52]. Less commonly reported are deep and superficial infections, hematoma, and fractures. The main variable that allows for a drastic reduction of complications is patient selection.

6.2.5   Discussion (Table 6.12)

Studies about DFO are all represented by small patient cohorts and low level of evidence, but all report agreement in improvements in arthritic pain. Other results are not well defined. Distal femoral osteotomy may allow an easier future knee replacement. The most performed v is the medial closing

Table 6.13 Opening wedge DFO

References	Year	Cases	Average age (years)	Mean follow-up	Fixation	Results	Complications	Range of motion	Angle HKS
Nicolaides et al. [70]	2000 Knee	2	20/44	1.3/1.1	Coralline wedge Cast	Good	None	Not reported	Preop 16° and 14° valgus Postop not reported
Puddu et al. [44]	2007 Sports Med Arthrosc Rev	21	54	from 4 to 14	Puddu plate	Improving in IKDC HSS from 60 to 87 points	Not reported	Not reported	Not reported
Das et al. [67]	2008 Open Acces Surg	12	34 (11–49)	6.1 (4.25–7.4)	Puddu plate	Lysholm from 64 to 76 Clinical HSS from 42 to 64 Functional HSS from 58 to 67	Not major complications reported	Not reported	Preop 16° valgus (10–21° valgus) Postop 5° valgus (1–8° valgus)
Jacobi et al. [69]	2011 Arch Orthop Trauma	14	46 (28–63)	3.8 (2.2–5.3)	Tomofix	50 % of osteotomies healed at 3 months, 14 % at 6 months and the others at 9 months. Mean satisfaction index was 78 %. KOOS from 31 to 69	9 including 2 nonunion 1 fracture 86 % of patients complain about plate intolerance	Not reported	Not reported
Zarrouck et al. [43]	2010 Orthop Traumatol Surg Res	22	53 (27–66)	4.5 (3–11)	90° blade plate	IKSS from 49.28 to 74.23 Functional score from 50.68 to 72.85	None	Not reported	Preop: 14.5° valgus (8–18° valgus) Postop: 5.5° valgus (3° varus–6° valgus)
Thein et al. [66]	2012 J Ortho	6	46.7	6.5	Puddu plate	Mean Oxford Knee Score from 13.1 to 26 Average subjective satisfaction rate 6.6 (at last fu on a scale of 0–10)	No major complications	Not reported	Preop 13.5° valgus mean Last fu 1.6° valgus mean

Author	Year/Journal	n	Mean age	Follow-up	Implant	Outcome	Complications	ROM	Alignment
Dewilde et al. [65]	2013 Knee Surg Sports Traumatol Arthrosc	16	47 (30–51)	5.6 (2.5–10.5)	Puddu plate	Average knee score from 43 preoperatively to 78 at last fu. Kellgreen-Lawrence osteoarthritis remained unchanged. Survivorship at 7 years fu 82 %	1 fracture	Not reported	Preop 6.5 valgus (3–10° valgus) Last fu 1.2° varus mean
Saithna et al. [68]	2014 Knee	21	41 (8–58)	4.5 (1.6–9.2)	Puddu plate Tomofix	The cumulative survival rate of 79 % at 5 years, with a significant improvement in all the outcomes evaluated (KOOS; IKDC; Lysholm-Tegner)	6 including 1 nonunion 2 losses of correction 1 infection	Not reported	% from medial to lateral Preop 75 % Last fu 37 %
Madelaine et al. [64]	2014 Knee Surg Sports Traumatol Arthrosc	29	44.4	6.66	95° blade plate	KSS from 80.5 to 65.8 Functional score from 50.4 to 68.5 Survivorship 91.4 % at 60 months	4 including 1 nonunion and 1 fracture	From 128.9° to 127.7°	Preop 7.8 valgus Last fu 0.4 valgus
Cameron et al. [71]	2014 Clin Orthop Relat Res	38 Arthritis group (61 %) Joint preservation group (39 %)	Not reported	5 (2–12)	22 Dynafix 6 Puddu plate 1 Tomofix	Joint preservation group: IKDC from 36 to 62. Survivorship at 5 years 92 % Arthritis group: IKDC from 47 to 67. Survivorship at 5 years 74 %	1 nonunion	Not reported	Joint preservation group: from 5° valgus to 2° varus Arthritis group: from 7° valgus to 2° varus

Table 6.14 Closing wedge DFO

References	Year	Cases	Average age (years old)	Mean follow-up (years)	Fixation	Results	Complications	Range of motion	Angle HKS
Johnson and Bodell [59]	1981 Mayo Clinic Proc	46	49 (17–76)	3.6	V blade plate or Steinmann pins or Harris splint or Kirschner wires or staple	22 good 15 fair 16 poor	Plate: 1 infection, 4 nonunions, 2 failure fixation Staples: 2 nonunion 2 failure fixation Pins: 1 nonunion	Not reported	Not reported
McDermott et al. [15]	1988 JBJS Am	24	53 (22–74)	4 (2–11.5)	90° blade plate	20/22 good results Improvement of 28 points in knee rating scale	1 failure fixation 1 superficial wound infection	Not reported	Not reported
Healy et al. [56]	1988 JBJS Am	23	56 (19–70)	4 (2–9)	90° blade plate	86 % were rated as good or excellent HSS score, from 65 to 86	2 nonunions 1 fracture	Not reported	Preop: 18° valgus mean Postop: 2° varus to 6° valgus
Learmonth [60]	1990 JBJS Br	12	40	3.5	90° blade plate	Good improving of pain	None	Not reported	Not reported
Edgerton et al. [52]	1993 Clin Orthop Rel Res	23	55	8.3	90° blade plate	Satisfactory results 71 %	17 including 7 delayed-nonunion	Not reported	Preop 18° valgus mean Postop 1° valgus mean
Finkelstein et al. [53]	1996 JBJS Am	21	56.3 (27–77)	11.1 (8.1–20)	90° blade plate	Average improvement in score of 30 points Survival rate 83 % at 40 months and 64 % at the final fu Survivorship at 10 years 64 %	7 including 1 femoral fracture and 1 loss of correction	Not reported	Last fu: 2° valgus mean
Cameron et al. [42]	1997 Can J Surg	49	60 (23–84)	3.5 (1–7)	90° blade plate	KSS postoperatively 84.8	1 loss of fixation 1 fracture	Not reported	Preop 13° valgus (7–23° valgus) Postop not reported

Mathews et al. [47]	1998 Orthopedics	21	53 (21–77)	3 (1–8)	10 cast 5 staple 6 AO blade plate	33 % of patients had a satisfactory result. HSS score from 61 to 64	57 % percent had significant complications including 1 wound infection 1 infected nonunion 4 nonunions and 11 implant failure	Not reported	Preop 14.7° valgus (6–32° valgus) Postop 5.1° valgus (0–20° valgus)
Stahelin et al. [45]	2000 JBJS AM	21	57 (39–71)	5 (2–12)	Semitubular AO plate	Average HSS score increased from 65 to 84 11 knees rated as excellent, 88 knees good	1 nonunion	No loss of ROM	Preop: 12° valgus (10–16° valgus) Last fu: 1.2° valgus (0–4° valgus)
Gross and Hutcjison [63]	2000 Oper Tech Sports Med	24	56 (27–77)	11.16 (5–20)	90° blade plate	Survivorship at 4 years 83 % and good functional results in 92 % Survivorship at 10 years 64 %	7 complications including 1 failure fixation 1 infection	Not reported	Not reported
Aglietti et al. [59]	2003 Am J Knee Surg	18	54 (38–75)	9	90° blade plate	77 % of good or excellent results	No patients had nonunion or infection. 3 loss of correction	Postop: 119° (95–135°)	Preop 11.5° valgus (5–18° valgus) Postop 1° valgus (5° varus–10° valgus)

(continued)

Table 6.14 (continued)

References	Year	Cases	Average age (years old)	Mean follow-up (years)	Fixation	Results	Complications	Range of motion	Angle HKS
Marin Morales et al. [50]	2000 Acta Orthop Belg	17	55 (50–72)	6.5 (2–15)	95° AO blade plate and straight blade plate	26.4 % excellent results 47.22 % good results HSS from 47.5 to 83.3	1 deep infection	Not reported	Preop 16° valgus (10–27° valgus) Last fu 1° valgus (10° varus–8° valgus)
Wang and Hsu [46]	2005 JBJS AM	30	53 (31–64)	8.3 (5.1–14.1)	90° blade plate	83 % satisfactory result KSS improved from 46 points to 88 points Survival rate at 10 years was 87 %	1 nonunion 1 fracture 2 losses of correction	From 121° (80–130°) to 124° (100–135°)	Preop 18.2° (12–27°) Last fu 1.2° valgus (6°-varus to 10° valgus)
Backstein et al. [38]	2007 J Arthroplast	38	44.1(20–67)	10.3 (3.3–20.4)	90° blade plate	60 % good or excellent results 10-year survival rate was 82 % Mean function HSS from 54 to 85.6	Not reported	Not reported	Preop 11.6° valgus (4–15 valgus) Postop 1.2° varus (0–5° varus)
Van Heerwaarden et al. [49]	2007 Oper Techn Orthop	59	37.5 (17–79.6)	Not reported	Tomofix	Not reported	2 losses of correction 1 infection	Not reported	Not reported
Omidi-Kashani et al. [57]	2009 J Orthop Surg Res	23	23.3(17–41)	1.3 (0.6–2.08)	90° blade plate	Mean knee score from 90.7 preoperatively to 98.13 at last fu	2 nonunions 1 wound infection	Referred no loss of knee motion	From 18° valgus to 2° valgus
Kosashvili et al. [55]	2010 Int Orthop	33	45.5 (24–63)	15.1 (10–25)	90° blade plate	58.8 % had good or excellent results in function score. Modified KSS from 36.8 to 60.2 (at last fu) Failure rate 48.5 % at 15.6 years	Not reported	Not reported	Not reported

Freiling et al. [61]	2010 Oper Orthop Traumatol	60	39.7 (17–79)	1.8 (0.2–3.8)	Tomofix	Tegner activity score from 2.8 to 5.6	3 delayed or nonunion	Preop 126° (95–140°) Postop 128° (105–140°)	Not reported
Sternheim et al. [58]	2011 Orthopedics	45	46.2 (24–67)	13.3 (3–25)	90° blade plate	Survivorship at 10-15-20 years was 90–79 %–21.5 % respectively Modified KSS from 36.1 to 60.5	Not reported	Not reported	Not reported
Petersen and Forkel [62]	2013 Oper Orthop Traumatol	23	Not reported	3.5	Angle-stable locking plate (LOQTEQ)	KOOS from 48.4 to 84.9	1 loss of correction	Not reported	Not reported
Forkel et al. [54]	2014 Knee Surg Sports Traumatol Arthrosc	22	47 (25–55)	1.13 (1–1.5)	Angle-stable locking plate	Increasing in all KOOS scores subgroups No difference in the two subgroup analysis: patients with and without microfracture and age (<50 vs. >50 years) Tegner from 3.5 to 4.2	1 loss of correction	Not reported	Not reported

wedge osteotomy which shows variable results from a 92 % of survivorship at 4 years follow-up to a 45 % of survivorship at 15 years follow-up. Technically, it is more difficult to perform than lateral opening wedge, which is probably why the lateral opening is preferred by some surgeons. Advantages are a more precise correction due to the gradual opening and the easier surgical approach. But it is associated with plate irritation that gives discomfort to the majority of patients and may be associated with slow bone healing. Perpendicular cuts give less stability than oblique cuts. For this reason, Jacobi et al. does not recommend lateral opening DFO even if patients were satisfied. It is important to perform thorough preoperative planning. There are some studies that compare medial closing to lateral opening DFO, and these studies reported good results with both techniques [73, 74, 76].

6.2.6   Conclusions

As reported in the literature, DFO provides an effective surgical treatment for unicompartmental arthritis associated with a valgus deformity in long-term follow-up. In addition, performing a DFO might provide easier terrain for a future TKA. Both techniques (medial closing or lateral opening) are valid and are effective in selected patients who wish to remain active.

6.3   Osteotomy around the Patellofemoral Joint

6.3.1   Introduction

Patellofemoral pain syndrome (PFPS), also described as an anterior knee pain, is a common reason for presentation to orthopedic surgeons. Trauma, overuse, and patellofemoral malalignment are more common causes of anterior knee pain in young adults and middle-aged patients [77, 78]. Chondromalacia patellae (Aleman 1917) is a softening of the articular cartilage, with an abnormal stress secondary to shear forces [79]. Isolated patellofemoral osteoarthritis (IPFOA) is a common disorder of multifactorial etiology but in many cases related to trochlear dysplasia

and disorders of patellar tilt and shift [80]. The optimum treatment for anterior knee pain associated with patellofemoral osteoarthritis remains controversial, and various surgical options have been proposed when there is a failure of conservative management which is up to 35 %, and relief of articular contact stress in the patellofemoral joint may be desirable when patellar articular surface is degenerating [79–82]. Different surgical treatments have been described for IPFOA: arthroscopic lavage and debridement, drilling or microfracture of the damaged surface, anterior elevation (Maquet) or anteromedialization of the tibial tubercle (Fulkerson), lateral retinacular release, partial lateral facetectomy of the patella, patellofemoral joint replacement, arthroplasty, and patellectomy [83].

1. The Maquet osteotomy (Maquet, 1976) aims to elevate the tibial tubercle 20–25 mm in one plane in order to increase the lever arm of the extensor mechanism (quadriceps tendon) and reduce the patellofemoral contact stresses [79, 82, 85–87]. Though attaining satisfactory clinical results with improvements in function and pain relief between 63 and 97 % of patients [87, 88], Maquet osteotomy is associated with major complications, and up to 40 % of patients were reported to have problems with delayed wound healing, tibial tubercle and proximal tibial fractures, and nonunion at the osteotomy sites [82, 85, 89]. This procedure has now generally been abandoned.

2. The origins of the "Fulkerson osteotomy" can be traced to Bandi [90] and Maquet [91] who demonstrated pain reduction in patients with painful patellofemoral arthrosis when the tibial tubercle was placed in a more anterior position. The Bandi-Maquet procedure decreases patellofemoral contact force and increases the patella moment arm by opening the angle between the quadriceps and patellar tendon. Thus patellofemoral joint reaction force is reduced on the diseased joint surface (typically distal patella), thereby reducing pain. John Fulkerson (1983) described a multiplane anteromedializing modification of the Elmslie-Trillat procedure that aims to decrease

the lateral facet contact pressures and realign the joint without the need for bone graft [92]. The indication for this operation is painful patellofemoral arthrosis, particularly when it is unipolar on the inferolateral patella facet [93]. This technique has reported good/excellent short-term clinical results in 60–90 % and an 84 % overall subjective improvement in symptoms. This technique also reported lower complication rates compared to the Maquet technique, although nonunion, loss of fixation, and tibial fractures have still occurred [82, 88, 89].

3. Partial lateral facetectomy is a simple, cost-effective surgical method that requires a short period of time for postoperative rehabilitation and allows a quick recovery with encouraging results. Its goal is to relieve symptoms but not to eliminate predisposing factors [83, 84].

The purpose of this section is to summarize the most common surgical techniques used for the treatment of IPFOA, highlighting surgical techniques, outcome, predictive factors, and complications of the most popular surgical techniques, Fulkerson and Maquet.

6.3.2 Surgical Techniques

6.3.2.1 Maquet Surgical Procedure

The skin is incised medial and parallel to the tibial crest below the anterior tuberosity. Using a Kirschner wire a series of parallel holes is drilled transversely 7–8 mm posterior to the tibial crest for a distance of 15 mm. The cleft outlined with the holes is completed by thin osteotome. The tibial crest is then lifted with the tibial tuberosity and the insertion of the patella tendon. A piece of iliac bone, 20–30 mm thick, is located proximally as possible, just beneath the anterior tuberosity. The skin suture may require two lateral relieving incisions when the forward displacement exceeds 2 cm [94]. The modified Maquet elevates the tibial tubercle 15–20 mm. Ferguson biomechanically analyzed anterior tibial tubercle advancement and reported that the first 10–15 mm of patellar tendon elevation reduced the average

stress in the joint by more than 80 %, lowering the complication rates [85, 95, 96].

6.3.2.2 Fulkerson Surgical Procedure

The anteromedialization osteotomy begins with an incision 5–6 cm in length, lateral to the tibial tubercle. The incision should be made large enough to limit damage to the skin and soft tissues. Dissection is continued to the level of the patella tendon insertion on the tibial tubercle. The anterior compartment musculature is exposed, then elevated from the lateral edge of the tibial crest, and retracted posteriorly to expose the posterior aspect of the tibia. Retractors are placed to expose the entire length of the planned osteotomy. The amount of medialization and anteriorization is determined by the obliquity of the osteotomy in the axial plane, with a more oblique (anterior to posterior) osteotomy producing more anteriorization for unloading of lateral and distal cartilaginous lesions. The osteotomy line is tapered to merge with the anterior tibial cortex at the most distal aspect of the osteotomy. The osteotomy cut is created using an oscillating saw from medial to lateral and anterior to posterior along the oblique axial plane. The cut should begin at the most distal aspect of the planned osteotomy and proceed proximally. An attempt should be made to leave a distal periosteal hinge along the tibial crest unless concomitant distalization is indicated. The oblique osteotomy is completed with an osteotome from lateral to medial just proximal to the patella tendon insertion on the tubercle to create a proximal bumper.

At this point, the osteotomized tubercle can be rotated anteriorly and medially along the oblique plane of the osteotomy. Temporary fixation of the tibial tubercle can be achieved. Special attention should be made to avoid overmedialization of extensor mechanism resulting in medial tracking. Typically, medialization greater than 1 cm is not recommended. Definitive fixation of the osteotomized fragment is achieved using 4.5 mm self-tapping screws. Screw placement is approximately 1 cm distal to the patella tendon insertion, and screws are spaced 2 cm apart to reduce the risk of fracture [92, 97, 98]. Some authors use a modification of Fulkerson technique with elevation of 1–1.5 cm [79] (Table 6.15).

Table 6.15 Advantages and disadvantages of anteromedialization

Advantages	Disadvantages
Preservation of the extensor mechanism	Fails to address incompetent MPFL
Large surface area for bone healing	Postoperative hardware irritation
Ability to place multiple screws	Potential neuromuscular injury
Multiplanar adjustments	Increased medial patellofemoral contact pressure
Early range of motions	Delayed union or nonunion
	Cannot be performed in skeletally immature

6.3.2.3 Partial Lateral Facetectomy Procedure

The knee is approached through a lateral parapatellar incision. A lateral retinacular release is done from the inferior to the superior pole of the patella. It is important not to injure the vastus lateralis. With the knee in extension, the patella and trochlear groove are observed for cartilage lesions and checked for patellofemoral congruency. About 1–1.5 cm of the lateral border of the patella, including osteophytes, and 1–2 mm of cartilage are resected with an oscillating saw. It has no detrimental effect on quadriceps function, but if the vastus lateralis is detached, complications such as medial patellar subluxation, patellar hypermobility, quadriceps weakness or rupture, hemarthrosis, and skin necrosis may occur. If a kissing lesion and osteophytes exist on the lateral condyle of the femur, they also are cut and trimmed. Range of motion and isometric quadriceps exercises are initiated as soon as possible, and weight-bearing is allowed in the first week postoperatively [83].

6.3.3 Results (Tables 6.16 and 6.17)

6.3.3.1 Outcomes

There are 15 published series of tibial tubercle osteotomy for patellofemoral osteoarthritis currently in the literature [77, 79, 81, 82, 86, 87, 93, 96, 99–105]. The studies were divided into two groups: the Maquet osteotomies (Table 6.16) and

Fulkerson osteotomies (Table 6.17). All the studies are retrospective except two [78, 87].

Combining the Maquet osteotomy and variations (modified Maquet and Ferguson osteotomy), the studies include 457 operated knees. Mean follow-up ranges from 17 to 192 months. There is a wide margin of the reported excellent/good results, which are between 10 and 100 %. Related to the Fulkerson osteotomy combined, the studies included 179 operated knees. Mean follow-up ranges from 28 to 72 months. There is an excellent/good result between 85.7 and 93 %.

6.3.3.2 Complications

Complication rates for Maquet osteotomy are between 13 and 38 %, mainly related to tibial fracture (especially tibial tubercle fracture and metaphyseal fracture), which represents 41 % of all complications (Table 6.16). Randin performed the initial Maquet osteotomy (20–25 mm of bone graft), modified Maquet (an elevation of 15–20 mm), and the Ferguson modification (10–15 mm) in order to compare the rate of complications [95]. Related to Fulkerson osteotomy, complication rates are between 0 and 33 %, mainly related to pain when kneeling because of which 26 % of patients required hardware removal.

6.3.4 Discussion

Chondromalacia patellae and patellofemoral osteoarthritis pose a difficult treatment problem for orthopedic surgeons. The initial treatment should be a nonoperative regimen, but some patients will subsequently require operative intervention for pain relief and functional improvement. Maquet osteotomy reported good results but with a high rate of complications and therefore is now rarely used. The Fulkerson method is now more commonly used, particularly to treat inferolateral patellar wear associated with malalignment in younger patients.

Apart from surgical technique, other variables are important, including patient selection and management of the soft tissues, which have

Table 6.16 Systematic review ATT osteotomies (Maquet)

Author	Year	Average age	Cohort (operated knees)	Outerbridge grade	Performed surgery	Follow-up (months)	Results	Complication rates	Complication
Lund et al. [27]	1980	34 (33–35)	68	I 22 %, II 17 %, III 38 %, IV 22 %	M	17 months	17 months, 70 % improvement (68 % men, average age: 27 years). 30 % no improvement (75 % women, average age: 37 years)	32 %	Skin necrosis 8, nerve palsy 3, tibial fracture 4, thrombosis 2, quadriceps rupture 1, DVT 1, granuloma 2, compartmental syndrome 1
Radin [21]	1986	29 (16–56)	54	–	M 22 %, MM 59 %, FM 16 %	24 months	M 91 % S/8.3 % F, MM 93 % S/6.3 % F, FM 66 % S/33.3 % F	M 41.7 %, MM 15.6 %, FM 22.2 %	–
Bessette et al. [24]	1986	34 (15–61)	21	–	MM	29 months	Not significative for: age, patella dislocations, crepitus, and ROM	38 %	Delayed skin healing 2, tibial fracture 2, delayed union 1, transfusion required 1, manipulation required 1, re-arthroscopy 1
Radin et al. [21]	1993	31 (16–49)	42	–	MM	144 months	OAP 86 % excellent/good, OARL 75 % excellent/good, OAPP 55 % good. Results not related to age, gender, follow up, during symptoms, cartilage damage	28 %	Nonunion 2, osteomyelitis 1, tibial fracture 9
Schmid [20]	1992	34 (20–66)	35	–	M 37.1 %, MM 28.6 %, FM 34.3 %	192 months	M 100 % excellent/good, MM 80 % excellent/good, FM 58 % excellent/good	–	–

(continued)

Table 6.16 (continued)

Author	Year	Average age	Cohort (operated knees)	Outerbridge grade	Performed surgery	Follow-up (months)	Results	Complication rates	Complication
Jenny et al. [19]	1996	43 (17–64)	100	I 15 %, II 16 %, III 21 %, IV 48 %	MM	48 months (100 %), 132 (96–180) months (65 %)	48 months 62 % good, 11 months 61 % good results not related to sex, age, weight. Only PF chondral lesion has predictive value	–	–
Rozbruch et al. [29]	1979	34	30	–	M	30 months	18 % excellent/good	27 %	Wound complications 4, infections 2, tibial fracture 2
Sudmann et al. [30]	1980	30	32	–	M	22 months	30 % excellent/good	18 %	Infections 2, others 2
Healtey et al. [31]	1984	53 (10–71)	29	–	M	36 months	19 % excellent/good	13 %	Infections 1, tibial fracture 3
Engebretsen et al. [32]	1989	39 (23–55)	46	–	M	60 months	10 % excellent/good	17 %	Infections 1, tibial fracture 1, others 6

Abbreviations: M Maquet, *MM* modified Maquet, *FM* Ferguson modification, *OAP* osteoarthritis post-traumatic, *OARL* osteoarthrosis post-recurrent subluxation, *OAPP* osteoarthrosis post- patelectomy, *PF* patellofemoral, *DVT* deep venous thrombosis

Table 6.17 Systematic review ATT osteotomies (Fulkerson)

Author	Year	Average age (years)	Cohort (operated knees)	Outerbridge grade	Performed surgery	Follow-up (months)	Results	Complication rates	Complication
Jack et al. [25]	2012	34.4 (19.6–52.2)	50	–	MF	72.4 months (62–118) 92 %	Kujala score improvement 67 % VAS improvement 36 % excellent/good 72 % procedure again 86 % significant differences in age but independent for chondromalacia	6 %	Tibial fracture 1, infection 1, others 1, knee pain with screw removal 6 (12)
Fulkerson et al. [4]	1990	28 (16–56)	51	–	F	35 months (26–50)	Final follow-up: subjective, 93 % excellent/good; objective, 89 % excellent/good	29 %	Stiffness 9, tibial tubercle fracture 2, DVT 2, weakness 2
Pidoriano et al. [13]	1997	29 (16–54)	37	I 75 %, II 80 %, III 64 %, IV 72 %	F	46.8 months (12–96)	DPOA 90 % excellent/good, LFOA 84 % excellent/good, MFOA 55 % excellent/good, PDOA 20 % 92 % would have the procedure again	8 %	Tibial fracture 1, wound dehiscence 1, arthrofibrosis 1, screw removal 27 (75 %)
Karamehmetoglu et al. [1]	2007	28.6 (21–42)	21	III–IV 100 %	F	28 months (20–60)	85.7 % excellent/good, EVA improvement: 53 %	33 %	Tibial tubercle avulsion 1, DVT 1, infection 1, flexion contracture 4, screw removal 15 (71.4 %)

(continued)

Table 6.17 (continued)

Author	Year	Average age (years)	Cohort (operated knees)	Outerbridge grade	Performed surgery	Follow-up (months)	Results	Complication rates	Complication
Atkinson et al. [7]	2009	27 (18–37)	20	Mean: 3.44. 100 % chondral damage on the lateral facet and distal patella	F	62 months (26–151)	EVA improvement, 44.4 %; S&T score improvement, 45.85 %	0 %	–

Abbreviations: DVT deep venous thrombosis, *F* Fulkerson, *MF* Fulkerson modification, *DPOA* distal patellar osteoarthrosis, *LFOA* lateral facet osteoarthrosis, *MFOA* medial facet osteoarthrosis, *PDOA* proximal or diffuse osteoarthrosis, *S&T score* Shelbourne and Trumper score a role in limiting complications. Age, weight, and gender have no proven predictive values [87, 96, 106].

Some authors reported better prognosis in "end-stage" cases (Outerbridge III–IV or Iwano grades II, III, and IV). Pidoriano [93] noted an improved activity level after anteromedial tibial tubercle transfer if a lateral or distal articular lesion is present. Patients with medial or proximal lesions, however, may not achieve satisfactory improvement in physical activity. Trochlear lesions were described at the time of surgery, reporting excellent/good results for lateral lesions and worse results for central lesions which are associated with lateral and medial patella lesions, respectively.

Partial lateral facetectomy, with or without a lateral retinacular release or lengthening, is a useful operation for advanced isolated patellofemoral arthrosis. Associated tibiofemoral arthritis, even when patellofemoral arthritis is most prominent, leads to poorer outcomes [80, 83, 107–109]. Isolated lateral retinacular release (LRR) alone has been shown to improve middle-aged and elderly patients with normal tibiofemoral alignment and joint, normal Q angle (<25°), and no lateral patellar subluxation on axial view [110]. LRR is reserved for patients with abnormal patellar tilt and no arthrosis. Patients with patellofemoral arthritis associated with lateral subluxation and lateral osteophytes have satisfaction rates between 88 and 90 % when lateral facetectomy is performed, with or without a lateral release, recognizing that a lateral facetectomy alone will relax the lateral structures [80, 83, 107–109].

Parvizi added that IPFOA had an increased prevalence of extensor mechanism malalignment and an increased requirement for LRR. Wetzels and Bellemans reported that the lateral release was necessary in 78.6 % of the 168 knees undergoing lateral facetectomy [84]. Paulos reported results of lateral facetectomy associated with LRR in 66 end-stage knees, with 88 % satisfied or very satisfied in 5 years mean follow-up [107]. Martens performed isolated lateral patellectomy in 20 knees and reported 65 % of good results and 25 % of moderate results at 2 year

follow-up. In long-term follow-up, Kaplan-Meier survival rates with reoperation as an end point were 85 % at 5 years, 67.2 % at 10 years, and 46.7 % at 20 years [84].

Isolated PFOA can also be treated by patellofemoral arthroplasty or TKA, although it is usually reserved for older patients. The success rate of patellofemoral arthroplasty varies from 44 to 90 %. Laskin reported that TKA for isolated PFOA provided excellent pain relief and improvement of function in 70–85 % [83].

6.3.5 Conclusion

Tibial tubercle anteromedialization osteotomy is an effective treatment for anterior knee pain. It can provide excellent/good long-term functional results in the majority of patients, with a very high grade of satisfaction levels and sustained improvement in pain. Knees with patellofemoral malalignment may benefit from an individualized medialization of the tibial tubercle. Lateral patellar facetectomy with or without formal LRR may also have high rates of satisfaction in longer term results.

6.4 Conclusions

Osteotomy around the knee joint is a particularly valuable procedure for a specific group of patients, as discussed in detail in this chapter. It is especially valuable in the management of OA in the younger patient, as it allows a significant improvement in pain and function without resorting to the irreversible arthroplasty option. It has also been shown to have a positive influence on the natural history of OA. Achieving success with osteotomy relies on careful patient selection, careful and precise surgical technique, and appropriately prescribed rehabilitation. If these requirements are met, then there is usually a significant, sustained improvement, and therefore all orthopedic surgeons managing these patients should be familiar and comfortable with the techniques described in this chapter.

6.5   Case Examples

Medial Opening HTO
Young active male, 45 years old, 180 cm, 105 kg,
previous medial meniscectomy 20 years ago

Suffers from medial pain during sport activities, and occasional pain when walking

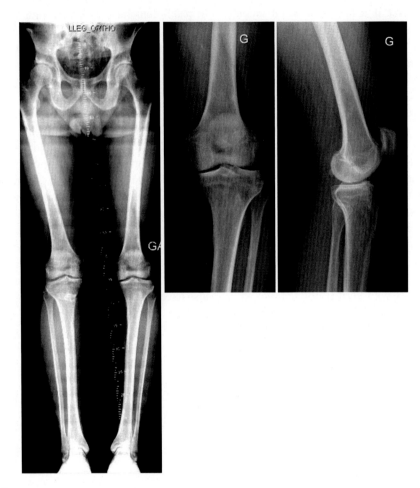

Preoperative

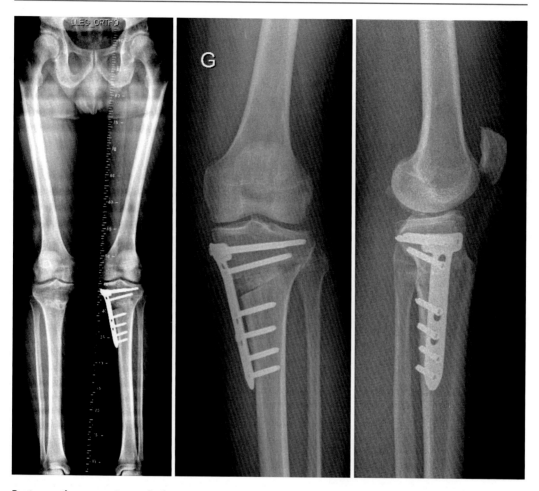

Postoperative x-rays, 2 months fu

Lateral closing HTO

Young active patient, 35 years old, ACL reconstruction and medial meniscectomy 15 years ago

Suffers from medial pain during daily activities

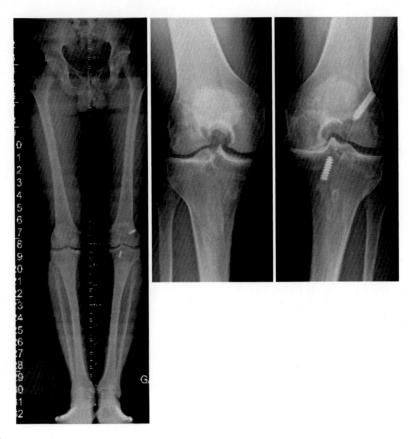

Preoperative

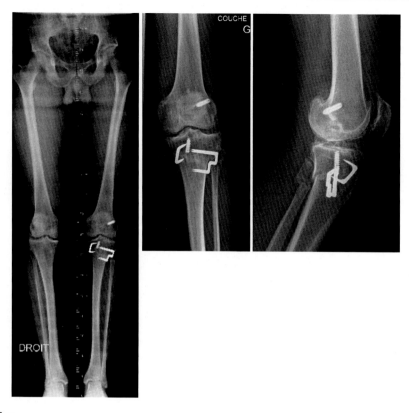

Postoperative

Lateral Opening DFO

Middle-aged female, 50 years old, previous lateral meniscectomy 15 years ago

Suffers from lateral knee pain, during daily activities

Preoperative

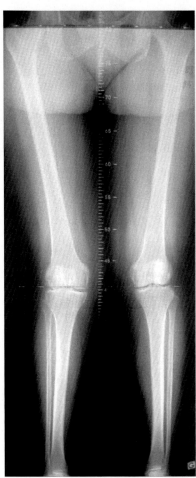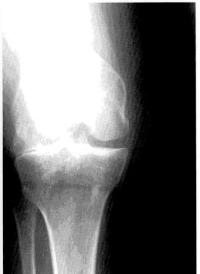

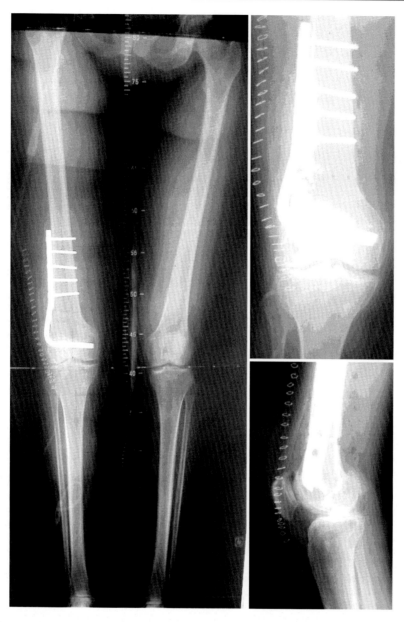

Postoperative

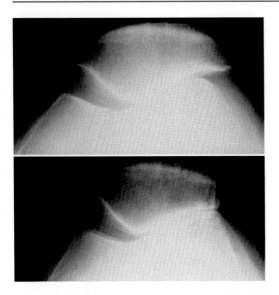

Lateral facetectomy

Acknowledgment We would like to acknowledge Professor Elisabeth Arendt for her help regarding the patellofemoral chapter.

References

1. Jackson JP, Waugh W. Tibial osteotomy for osteoarthritis of the knee. J Bone Joint Surg Br. 1961;43:746–51.
2. Gariepy R. Genu varum treated by high tibial osteotomy. J Bone Joint Surg Br. 1964;46:783–4.
3. Hernigou P, Medevielle D, Debeyre J, Goutallier D. Proximal tibial osteotomy for osteoarthritis with varus deformity. A ten to thirteen-year follow-up study. J Bone Joint Surg Am. 1987;69(3):332–54.
4. Debeyre J, Patte D. Intéret des ostéotomies de correction dans le traitement de certain gonarthroses avec déviation axiale. Rev Rhum Mal Osteoartic. 1962;29:722–9.
5. Maquet PGJ. Biomechanics of the knee: with application to the pathogenesis and the surgical treatment of osteoarthritis. 2nd ed. New York: Springer; 1984.
6. Aglietti P, Buzzi R, Vena LM, Baldini A, Mondaini A. High tibial valgus osteotomy for medial gonarthrosis: a 10- to 21-year study. J Knee Surg. 2003; 16(1):21–6.
7. Sprenger TR, Doerzbacher JF. Tibial osteotomy for the treatment of varus gonarthrosis. Survival and failure analysis to twenty-two years. J Bone Joint Surg Am. 2003;85-A(5):912.
8. Lash NJ, Feller JA, Batty LM, Wasiak J, Richmond AK. Bone grafts and bone substitutes for opening-wedge osteotomies of the knee: a systematic review. Arthroscopy. 2015;31(4):720–30.
9. Saragaglia D, Blaysat M, Inman D, Mercier N. Outcome of opening wedge high tibial osteotomy augmented with a Biosorb wedge and fixed with a plate and screws in 124 patients with a mean of ten years follow-up. Int Orthop. 2010;5:1151–6.
10. Flecher X, Parratte S, Aubaniac JM, Argenson JN. A 12-28-year follow-up study of closing wedge high tibial osteotomy. Clin Orthop Relat Res. 2006;452:91–6.
11. Benzakour T, Hefti A, Lemseffer M, El Ahmadi JD, Bouyarmane H, Benzakour A. High tibial osteotomy for medial osteoarthritis of the knee: 15 years follow-up. Int Orthop. 2010;34(2):209–15.
12. Majima T, Yasuda K, Katsuragi R, Kaneda K. Progression of joint arthrosis 10 to 15 years after high tibial osteotomy. Clin Orthop Relat Res. 2000;381:177–84.
13. Amendola A, Bonasia DE. Results of high tibial osteotomy: review of the literature. Int Orthop. 2010;34(2):155–60.
14. Brouwer RW, Huizinga MR, Duivenvoorden T, van Raaij TM, Verhagen AP, Bierma-Zeinstra SM, Verhaar JA. Osteotomy for treating knee osteoarthritis. Cochrane Database Syst Rev. 2014;12:CD004019.
15. McDermott PA, Finkelstein JA, Farine I, et al. Distal femoral varus osteotomy for valgus deformity of the knee. J Bone Joint Surg Am. 1988;70:110–6.
16. Marti RK, Verhagen RA, Kerkhoffs GM, Moojen TM. Proximal tibial varus osteotomy. Indications, technique, and five to twenty-one-year results. J Bone Joint Surg Am. 2001;83-A(2):164–70.
17. Arthur A, LaPrade RF, Agel J. Proximal tibial opening wedge osteotomy as the initial treatment for chronic posterolateral corner deficiency in the varus knee: a prospective clinical study. Am J Sports Med. 2007;35(11):1844–50.
18. Lustig S, Servien E, Demey G, Neyret P. Osteotomy for the arthritic knee: a European perspective. In: Scott WN (ed). Insall and Scott. Surgery of the Knee 5th edition. Churchill Livingstone Elservier; 2012.
19. Noyes FR. Opening wedge tibial osteotomy: the 3-triangle method to correct axial alignment and tibial slope. Am J Sports Med. 2005;33(3): 378–87.
20. Gstöttner M, Pedross F, Liebensteiner M, Bach C. Long-term outcome after high tibial osteotomy. Arch Orthop Trauma Surg. 2008;128(1):111–5.
21. Papachristou G, Plessas S, Sourlas J, Levidiotis C, Chronopoulos E, Papachristou C. Deterioration of long-term results following high tibial osteotomy in patients under 60 years of age. Int Orthop. 2006;30(5):403–8.
22. Koshino T, Yoshida T, Ara Y, Saito I, Saito T. Fifteen to twenty-eight years follow-up results of high tibial valgus osteotomy for osteoarthritic knee. Knee. 2004;11(6):439–44.
23. Hernigou P, Roussignol X, Flouzat-Lachaniette CH, Filippini P, Guissou I, Poignard A. Opening wedge tibial osteotomy for large varus deformity with Ceraver resorbable beta tricalcium phosphate wedges. Int Orthop. 2010;34(2):191–9.

24. Hernigou P, Ma W. Open wedge tibial osteotomy with acrylic bone cement as bone substitute. Knee. 2001;8(2):103–10.

25. Naudie D, Bourne RB, Rorabeck CH, Bourne TJ. The Install Award. Survivorship of the high tibial valgus osteotomy. A 10- to –22-year followup study. Clin Orthop Relat Res. 1999;367:18–27.

26. Yasuda K, Majima T, Tsuchida T, Kaneda K. A ten- to 15-year follow-up observation of high tibial osteotomy in medial compartment osteoarthrosis. Clin Orthop Relat Res. 1992;282:186–95.

27. Yasuda K, Majima T, Tanabe Y, Kaneda K. Long-term evaluation of high tibial osteotomy for medial osteoarthritis of the knee. Bull Hosp Jt Dis Orthop Inst. 1991;51(2):236–48.

28. Ivarsson I, Myrnerts R, Gillquist J. High tibial osteotomy for medial osteoarthritis of the knee. A 5 to 7 and 11 year follow-up. J Bone Joint Surg Br. 1990;72(2):238–44.

29. Schallberger A. High tibial valgus osteotomy in unicompartmental medial osteoarthritis of the knee: a retrospective follow-up study over 13–21 years. Knee Surg Sports Traumatol Arthrosc. 2011;19(1):122–7.

30. Akizuki S, Shibakawa A, Takizawa T, Yamazaki I, Horiuchi H. The long-term outcome of high tibial osteotomy: a ten- to 20-year follow up. J Bone Joint Surg Br. 2008;90:592–6.

31. Babis GC, An KN, Chao EY, Larson DR, Rand JA, Sim FH. Upper tibia osteotomy: long term results – realignment analysis using OASIS computer software. J Orthop Sci. 2008;13(4):328–34.

32. Omori G, Koga Y, Miyao M, Takemae T, Sato T, Yamagiwa H. High tibial osteotomy using two threaded pins and figure-of-eight wiring fixation for medial knee osteoarthritis: 14 to 24 years follow-up results. J Orthop Sci. 2008;13(1):39–45. 2008 Feb 16.

33. Howells NR, Salmon L, Waller A, Scanelli J, Pinczewski LA. The outcome at ten years of lateral closing-wedge high tibial osteotomy: determinants of survival and functional outcome. Bone Joint J. 2014;96-B(11):1491–7.

34. Aoki Y, Yasuda K, Mikami S, Ohmoto H, Majima T, Minami A. Inverted V-shaped high tibial osteotomy compared with closing-wedge high tibial osteotomy for osteoarthritis of the knee. Ten-year follow-up result. J Bone Joint Surg Br. 2006;88(10):1336–40.

35. van Raaij T, Reijman M, Brouwer RW, Jakma TS, Verhaar JN. Survival of closing-wedge high tibial osteotomy: good outcome in men with low-grade osteoarthritis after 10–16 years. Acta Orthop. 2008;79(2):230–4.

36. El-Azab H, et al. The effect of closed- and open-wedge high tibial osteotomy on tibial slope. A retrospective radiological review of 120 cases. JBJS (Br). 2008;90-B(9):1193–7.

37. Tigani D, Ferrari D, Trentani P, Barbanti-Brodano G, Trentani F. Patellar height after high tibial osteotomy. Int Orthop. 2001;24(6):331–4.

38. Backstein D, Morag G, Hanna S, Safir O, Gross A. Long- term follow-up of distal femoral varus osteotomy of the knee. J Arthroplasty. 2007;22:2–6.

39. Haviv B, Bronak S, Thein R, Thein R. The results of corrective osteotomy for valgus arthritic knees. Knee Surg Sports Traumatol Arthrosc. 2013;21:49–56.

40. Rosso F, Margheritini F. Distal femoral osteotomy. Curr Rev Musculoskelet Med. 2014;7(4):302–11.

41. W-Dahl A, Lidgren L, Sundberg M, Robertsson O. Introducing prospective national registration of knee osteotomies. A report from the first year in Sweden. Int Orthop. 2014(Dec 14).

42. Cameron HU, Botsford DJ, Park YS. Prognostic factors in the outcome of supracondylar femoral osteotomy for lateral compartment osteoarthritis of the knee. Can J Surg. 1997;2:114–8.

43. Zarrouk A, Bouzidi R, Karray B, Kammoun S, Mourali S, Kooli M. Distal femoral varus osteotomy outcome: is associated femoropatellar osteoarthritis consequential? Orthop Traumatol Surg Res. 2010;96:632–6.

44. Puddu G, Cipolla M, Cerullo G, Franco V, Giannì E. Osteotomies: the surgical treatment of the valgus knee. Sports Med Arthrosc. 2007;15(1):15–22.

45. Stahelin T, Hardegger F, Ward JC. Supracondylar osteotomy of the femur with use of compression. Osteosynthesis with a malleable implant. J Bone Joint Surg Am. 2000;82(5):712–22.

46. Wang J-W, Hsu C-C. Distal femoral varus osteotomy for osteoarthritis of the knee. J Bone Joint Surg Am. 2005;87:127–33.

47. Mathews J, Cobb AG, Richardson S, Bentley G. Distal femoral osteotomy for lateral compartment osteoarthritis of the knee. Orthopedics. 1998;21(4):437–40.

48. Puddu GCM, Cerullo G, Franco V, Giannì E. Which osteotomy for a valgus knee? Int Orthop. 2010;34(2):239–47.

49. Van Heerwaarden R, Wymenga A, Freiling D, et al. Distal medial closed wedge varus femur osteotomy stabilized with the Tomofix plate fixator. Oper Techn Orthop. 2007;17(1):12–21.

50. Marin Morales LA, Gomez Navalon LA, Zorrilla Ribot P, Salido Valle JA. Treatment of osteoarthritis of the knee with val- gus deformity by means of varus osteotomy. Acta Orthop Belg. 2000;66:272–8.

51. Aglietti P, Menchetti PP. Distal femoral varus osteotomy in the valgus osteoarthritis knee. Am J Knee Surg. 2000;13:89–95.

52. Edgerton BC, Mariani EM, Morrey BF. Distal femoral varus osteotomy for painful genu valgum. A five-to-11-year follow-up study. Clin Orthop Relat Res. 1993;288:263–9.

53. Finkelstein JA, Gross AE, Davis A. Varus osteotomy of the distal part of the femur. A survivorship analysis. J Bone Joint Surg Am. 1996;78:1348–52.

54. Forkel P, Achtnich A, Metzlaff S, Zantop T, Petersen W. Midterm results following medial closed wedge distal femoral osteotomy stabilized with a locking internal fixation device. Knee Surg Sports Traumatol Arthrosc. 2014(Mar 28).

55. Kosashvili Y, Safir O, Gross A, Morag G, Lakstein D, Backstein D. Distal femoral varus osteotomy for lateral osteoarthritis of the knee: a minimum ten-year follow-up. Int Orthop. 2010;34:249–54.

56. Healy WL, Anglen JO, Wasilewsky SA, et al. Distal femoral varus osteotomy. J Bone Joint Surg Am. 1988;70:102–9.

57. Omidi-Kashani F, Hasankhani IG, Mazlumi M, Ebrahimzadeh MH. Varus distal femoral osteotomy in young adults with valgus knee. J Orthop Surg Res. 2009;4:15.

58. Sternheim A, Garbedian S, Backstein D. Distal femoral varus osteotomy: unloading the lateral compartment: long-term follow-up of 45 medial closing wedge osteotomies. Orthopedics. 2011;34:e488–90.

59. Johnson Jr EW, Bodell LS. Corrective supracondylar osteotomy for painful genu valgum. Mayo Clin Proc. 1981;56(2):87–92.

60. Learmonth ID. A simple technique for varus supra-condylar osteotomy in genu valgum. J Bone Joint Surg Br. 1990;72(2):235–7.

61. Freiling D, van Heerwaarden R, Staubli A, Lobenhoffer P. The medial closed-wedge osteotomy of the distal femur for the treatment of unicompart-mental lateral osteoarthritis of the knee. Oper Orthop Traumatol. 2010;22(3):317–34.

62. Petersen W, Forkel P. Medial closing wedge osteotomy for correction of genu valgum and torsional malalign-ment. Oper Orthop Traumatol. 2013;25(6):593–607.

63. Gross A, Hutchison CR. Realignment osteotomy of the knee-Part 1: distal femoral varus osteotomy for osteoarthritis of the valgus knee. Oper Tech Sports Med. 2000;8(2):122–6.

64. Madelaine A, Lording T, Villa V, Lustig S, Servien E, Neyret P. The effect of lateral opening wedge dis-tal femoral osteotomy on leg length. Knee Surg Sports Traumatol Arthrosc. 2014(Oct 19).

65. Dewilde TR, Dauw J, Vandenneucker H, Bellemans J. Opening wedge distal femoral varus osteotomy using the Puddu plate and calcium phosphate bone cement. Knee Surg Sports Traumatol Arthrosc. 2013;21:249–54.

66. Thein R, Bronak S, Thein R, Haviv B. Distal femoral osteotomy for valgus arthritic knees. J Orthop Sci. 2012;17(6):745–9.

67. Das DH, Sijbesma T, Hoekstra H, van Leeuwen W. Distal femoral opening-wedge osteotomy for lat-eral compartment osteoarthritis of the knee. Open Access Surg. 2008;1:25–9.

68. Saithna A, Kundra R, Getgood A, Spalding T. Opening wedge distal femoral varus osteotomy for lateral compartment osteoarthritis in the valgus knee. Knee. 2014;21(1):172–5.

69. Jacobi M, Wahl P, Bouaicha S, Jakob RP, Gautier E. Distal femoral varus osteotomy: problems associ-ated with the lateral open-wedge technique. Arch Orthop Trauma Surg. 2011;131(6):725–8.

70. Nicolaides AP, Papanikolaou A, Polyzoides AJ. Successful treatment of valgus deformity of the knee with an open supra- condylar osteotomy using a

coral wedge: a brief report of two cases. Knee. 2000;7(2):105–7.

71. Cameron JI, McCauley JC, Kermanshahi AY, Bugbee WD. Lateral opening-wedge distal femoral osteotomy: pain relief, functional improvement, and survivorship at 5 years. Clin Orthop Relat Res. 2014(Dec 24).

72. Brinkman JM, Freiling D, Lobenhoffer P, Staubli AE, van Heerwaarden RJ. Supracondylar femur osteotomies around the knee: patient selection, plan-ning, operative techniques, stability of fixation, and bone healing. Orthopade. 2014;43 Suppl 1:S1–10.

73. Zilber S, Larrouy M, Sedel L, Nizard R. Distal femoral varus osteotomy for symptomatic genu valgum: long-term results and review of the literature. Rev Chir Orthop Reparatrice Appar Mot. 2004;90:659–65.

74. Terry GC, Cimino PM. Distal femoral osteotomy for valgus deformity of the knee. Orthopedics. 1992;15(11):1283–9; discussion 1289–90.

75. Sharma L, Song J, Felson DT, Cahue S, Shamiyeh E, Dunlop DD. The role of knee alignment in disease progression and functional decline in knee osteoar-thritis. JAMA. 2001;286(2):188–95.

76. Saragaglia D, Chedal-Bornu B. Computer-assisted osteotomy for valgus knees: medium-term results of 29 cases. Orthop Traumatol Surg Res. 2014;100(5):527–30.

77. Karamehmetoğlu M, Oztürkmen Y, Azboy I, Caniklioğlu M. Fulkerson osteotomy for the treat-ment of chronic patellofemoral malalignment. Acta Orthop Traumatol Turc. 2007;41(1):21–30.

78. Fulkerson JP. Diagnosis and treatment of patients with patellofemoral pain. Am J Sports Med. 2002;30(3):447–56.

79. Jack CM, et al. The modified tibial tubercle osteot-omy for anterior knee pain due to chondromalacia patellae in adults. A five-year perspective study. Bone Joint Res. 2012;1:167–73.

80. Montserrat F, Alentorn-Geli E, León V, Ginés-Cespedosa A, Rigol P. Partial lateral facetectomy plus Insall's procedure for the treatment of isolated patellofemoral osteoarthritis: survival analysis. Knee Surg Sports Traumatol Arthrosc. 2014;22(1):88–96.

81. Fulkerson JP, Becker GJ, Meaney JA, Miranda M, Folcik MA. Anteromedial tibial tubercle transfer without bone graft. Am J Sports Med. 1990;18(5):490–6; discussion 496–7.

82. Atkinson HD, Bailey CA, Anand S, Johal P, Oakeshott RD. Tibial tubercle advancement osteot-omy with bone allograft for patellofe moral arthritis: a retrospective cohort study of 50 knees. Arch Orthop Trauma Surg. 2012;132(4):437–45.

83. Yercan HS, Ait Si Selmi T, Neyret P. The treatment of patellofemoral osteoarthritis with partial lateral face-tectomy. Clin Orthop Relat Res. 2005;436:14–9.

84. Wetzels T, Bellemans J. Patellofemoral osteoarthritis treated by partial lateral facetectomy: results at long-term follow up. Knee. 2012;19(4):411–5.

85. Radin EL. The Maquet procedure: anterior displace-ment of the tibial tubercle. Indications,

contraindications, and precautions. Clin Orthop Relat Res. 1986;213:241–8.

86. Engebretsen L, Svenningsen S, Benum P. Advancement of the tibial tuberosity for patellar pain. A 5-year follow-up. Acta Orthop Scand. 1989; 60(1):20–2.

87. Bessette GC, Hunter RE. The Maquet procedure. A retrospective review. Clin Orthop Relat Res. 1988;(232):159–67.

88. Farr J, Schepsis A, Cole B, Fulkerson J, Lewis PJ. Anteromedialization: review and technique. Knee Surg. 2007;20(2):120–8.

89. Sherman SL, Erickson BJ, Cvetanovich GL, Chalmers PN, Farr 2nd J, Bach Jr BR, Cole BJ. Tibial tuberosity osteotomy: indications, techniques, and outcomes. Am J Sports Med. 2013;42(8):2006–17.

90. Bandi W. Chondromalacia patellae and femoropatellar arthrosis, etiology, clinical aspects and therapy. Helv Chir Acta. 1972;39 Suppl 11:11–70.

91. Maquet P. Advancement of the tibial tuberosity. Clin Orthop Relat Res. 1976;115:225–30.

92. Fulkerson JP. Anteromedialization of the tibial tuberosity for patellofemoral malalignement. Clin Orth Relat Res. 1983;177:176–81.

93. Pidoriano AJ, Weinstein RN, Buuck DA, Fulkerson JP. Correlation of patellar articular lesions with results from anteromedial tibial tubercle transfer. Am J Sports Med. 1997;25(4):533–7.

94. Maquet P. Mechanics and osteoarthritis of the patellofemoral joint. Clin Orthop Relat Res. 1979;144: 70–3.

95. Bellemans J, Cauwenberghs F, Brys P, Victor J, Fabry G. Fracture of the proximal tibia after Fulkerson anteromedial tibial tubercle transfer. A report of four cases. Am J Sports Med. 1998;26(2):300–2.

96. Radin EL, Pan HQ. Long-term follow-up study on the Maquet procedure with special reference to the causes of failure. Clin Orthop Relat Res. 1993; 290:253–8.

97. Post WR, Fulkerson JP. Distal realignment of the patellofemoral joint. Indications, effects, results, and recommendations. Orthop Clin North Am. 1992; 23(4):631–43.

98. Duchman K, Bollier M. Distal realignment: indications, technique, and results. Clin Sports Med. 2014;33(3):517–30.

99. Jenny JY, Sader Z, Henry A, Jenny G, Jaeger JH. Elevation of the tibial tubercle for patellofemoral pain syndrome. An 8- to 15-year follow-up. Knee Surg Sports Traumatol Arthrosc. 1996;4(2):92–6.

100. Schmid F. The Maquet procedure in the treatment of patellofemoral osteoarthrosis. Long-term results. Clin Orthop Relat Res. 1993;294:254–8.

101. Nguyen C, Rudan J, Simurda MA, Cooke TD. High tibial osteotomy compared with high tibial and Maquet procedures in medial and patellofemoral compartment osteoarthritis. Clin Orthop Relat Res. 1989;245:179–87.

102. Lund F. Anterior displacement of the tibial tuberosity in chondromalacia patellae. Acta Ortho Scan. 1980;51:679–88.

103. Rozbruch JD, Campbell RD, Insall J. Tibial tubercle elevation (the Maquet operation): a clinical study of 31 cases. Ortho Trans. 1979;3:291.

104. Sudmann E, Salkowisch B. Anterior displacement of the tibial tuberosity in chondromalacia patellae. Acta Orthop Scan. 1980;51:679.

105. Heatley FW, Allen PR, Patrick JH. Tibial tubercle advancement for anterior knee pain. A temporary or permanent solution. Clin Orthop Relat Res. 1986;208:215–24.

106. Rappoport L, Browne G. The Maquet osteotomy. Orthop Clin North Am. 1992;23(4):645–56.

107. Paulos LE, O'Connor DL, Karistinos A. Partial lateral patellar facetectomy for treatment of arthritis due to lateral patellar compression syndrome. Arthroscopy. 2008;24(5):547–53.

108. Aderinto J, Cobb AG. Lateral release for patellofemoral arthritis. Arthroscopy. 2002;18(4):399–403.

109. Martens M, De Rycke J. Facetectomy of the patella in patellofemoral osteoarthritis. Acta Orthop Belg. 1990;56(3–4):563–7.

110. Alemdaroglu KB, Cimen O, Aydogan NH, Atlihan D, Iltar S. Early results of arthroscopic lateral retinacular release in patellofemoral osteoarthritis. Knee. 2008;15(6):451–5.

Unicompartmental Knee Arthroplasty in the Young Patient

7

Travis Loidolt and Brian Curtin

Contents

T. Loidolt, DO, MBA
Department of Orthopedic Surgery, St. Anthony Hospital, Oklahoma City, OK, USA

B. Curtin, MD (✉)
Ortho Carolina, Charlotte, NC, USA
e-mail: bmcurt01@gmail.com

7.1 Introduction

Historically, advances in total knee arthroplasty (TKA) with regard to implant design and surgical technique have resulted in improved clinical outcomes and survivorship [1]. Despite the functional advantages of unicompartmental knee arthroplasty (UKA), advances in clinical outcomes and survivorship continue to be somewhat limited [2–5]. Proponents of UKA cite multiple advantages of UKA over TKA. These include accelerated patient rehabilitation and recovery, less blood loss, lower morbidity, and preservation of normal knee kinematics [6].

In the United States (US), there is a current trend in orthopedics to provide patients with minimally invasive surgery resulting in a speedy recovery. The interest in UKA has continued to increase at a rate triple that of TKA [7]. This is compounded for the working age population (45–64 years old), which has been expected to represent 1/3 of all arthroplasty cases by the year 2030 [8]. This is not

© ISAKOS 2016
D.A. Parker (ed.), *Management of Knee Osteoarthritis in the Younger, Active Patient: An Evidence-Based Practical Guide for Clinicians*, DOI 10.1007/978-3-662-48530-9_7

the case worldwide. For example, in Sweden, the use of UKA decreased by 8 % between 2012 and 2013 and accounted for only 4.1 % of the number of arthroplasty procedures performed in the country in 2013 [9]. Likewise, in Australia, UKA decreased 2.7 % between 2012 and 2013 and accounted for 9.9 % of primary knee procedures in 2013 [10]. The UK Joint Registry is on par with these registries with regard to UKA as a percentage of primary knee procedures (9.2 %) but showed only a 0.4 % decrease in this percentage between 2012 and 2013 [11]. There were 725 UKA procedures in the New Zealand Joint Registry, which accounted for 9.8 % of primary knee procedures and represented a decrease of 0.3 % between 2012 and 2013 [12]. Regardless of where the joint surgeon is located, UKA has the potential to be a significant portion of one's practice, and understanding of the current literature and treatment algorithms is imperative to a successful outcome.

7.2   Basic Design Principles

Successful UKA implant design relies on long-term fixation to host bone while optimizing contact area and limiting constraint between the components, which will result in decreased polyethylene wear and contact stress. Increased constraint can result in accelerated loosening and implant failure, which has been reported with such UKA designs. This is due to the main driver of the knee kinematics in UKA knees being the cruciate ligaments and un-resurfaced compartments, and as such, a fixed-bearing UKA cannot be fully conforming [13].

There has been some data in the past studies showing failure rates (end point being revision surgery) for UKA in young patients (<60 years old) as high as 72 % at 7 years [14]. It has been thought that the failures described in older studies are at least partially as a result of design flaws including metal-backed tibial poly components leading to rapid poly wear as well as issues with femoral component loosening at the cement–component interface [15]. One difficulty often found with reviewing the literature related to outcomes is that a prosthesis used may later be recalled or discontinued [16].

A study by Fehring et al. [17] looked at reasons for early failure in UKA over two separate periods of time: 1990–1999 (period 1) and 2000–2008 (period 2). The findings indicate that the early failure rate is on the rise; however, the reason for failure differed between period 1 and period 2 (poly wear and loosening vs. technical errors, respectively) and, as such, should serve as a reminder to thoroughly review the literature and understand the history of UKA designs.

7.3   Unicompartmental Knee Arthroplasty Indications

7.3.1   General

The indications for unicompartmental knee arthroplasty have somewhat expanded since first described by Kozinn and Scott [18]. The historical indications for unicompartmental knee arthroplasty have been:

1. Medial or lateral compartmental osteoarthritis or osteonecrosis
2. Age >60 years with a low activity level
3. Weight <82 kg
4. Minimal pain at rest
5. Range-of-motion (ROM) arc >90° with <5° flexion contracture
6. Angular deformity <15° that is passively correctable to neutral

Based on the above criteria, it has been shown that approx. 6 % of total joint patients will qualify for a UKA [19]. These criteria have subsequently been proven to provide excellent results (96 % survival at 13 years) in unicompartmental arthroplasty at a minimum of 10 years even when they were made to be less stringent (flexion contracture of <15° instead of <5°, a weight of <124.7 kg instead of <82 kg, and an age >50 years old instead of >60 years old) [20]. The following criteria (Table 7.1) are an initial screening tool to help the surgeon quickly rule out potential UKA candidates. These are further broken down into their compartment-specific criteria in the sections to follow.

Although there are restrictions with regard to BMI, it should be noted that a recent study

Table 7.1 Revised indication for UKA

Medial or lateral compartmental osteoarthritis or osteonecrosis
Age >50 years old
Weight <124.7 kg
Minimal pain at rest
Range-of-motion (ROM) arc >90° with <15° flexion contracture
Angular deformity <15° that is passively correctable to neutral

Table 7.2 Indications for a medial UKA [19, 25]

Unicompartmental involvement (Ahlback stage narrowing greater than or equal to 2)
100° ROM
Full extension
Absence of patellofemoral joint (PFJ) involvement 30°, 60°, 90° flexion views
Total correction of deformity in coronal plane on stress x-rays
Full-thickness cartilage in lateral compartment
Intact ACL (verified with MRI if needed) or ability of the surgeon to perform a reconstruction

showed no correlation between BMI and revision rates at 5 years [21]. Further research is warranted in this area.

In addition to the above physical exam findings, a thorough preoperative workup is necessary. Radiographs including a weight-bearing anteroposterior (AP), lateral, stress, and patellar views should be obtained to help determine whether the patient is an appropriate candidate for UKA.

7.3.2 Medial UKA

Recent literature regarding medial UKA (MUKA) has investigated additional criteria which have expanded the ideal patient to include the younger population as well as created some specific indications such as intact ACL and a deformity that corrects ≤10° for a varus knee and ≤5° in a valgus knee [22–24].

The recent literature has continued to emphasize that regardless of the patient's age, thorough preoperative evaluation is imperative. This includes thorough history and physical exam. With the strict inclusion criteria, a missed contraindication can have catastrophic results. The current trends that differ from the "older patient" criteria seem to favor full-thickness cartilage in the opposite compartment, intact ACL, and full extension (Table 7.2).

It is worth mentioning that there has been evidence against performing a MUKA in a knee with less than severe arthritic change. Niinimäki et al. [26] reported a series of 113 MUKAs with a mean follow-up of 63 months and examined the reoperation rates as they related to a number of factors. They determined that reoperation rates were dependent on the joint space preoperatively.

When the thickness of the medial joint space was >2 mm, the revision rate was six times higher and eight times higher when the medial space was >40 % of the thickness of the lateral space.

In summary, the criteria for MUKA are extremely rigid and require that a surgeon be well versed in patient selection to ensure proper preoperative discussions and consistent outcomes.

7.3.3 Lateral UKA

The indications for lateral UKA (LUKA) have been extrapolated from Kozinn and Scott [18] and narrowed. There is a lack of studies including younger patients. For example, Pennington et al. [27] and Smith et al. [28] reported an average age of 68 years old and 64.8 years old, respectively. Their indications were as follows:

1. Diagnosis of noninflammatory arthritis
2. At least 90° of knee flexion
3. Intact ACL
4. Flexion contracture of ≤10°
5. Maximum valgus deformity of 20° that can be corrected to <7° of valgus (with the knee in maximum extension)

Pennington et al. also included patients with arthrosis secondary to trauma, weight >180 lbs., and osteophytes or chondrocalcinosis seen on radiographs. The authors used intraoperative examination of the other two compartments in their decision-making process. If the uninvolved compartment and the patellofemoral joint contained

Table 7.3 Indications for PFA as described by Lonner [29]

<60 years old
Chondromalacia grade I or II
Q-Angle <20° in women and <15° in men (unless corrected prior to PFA with anteromedialization of the tibial tubercle)
Lack of medial or lateral joint line pain
Absence of patellofemoral maltracking or malalignment

Outerbridge grade 2 or less, they proceeded with LUKA.

The key to LUKA is understanding the mechanics of the lateral femoral condyle on the tibia as the knee progresses through its range of motion. Pennington et al. [27] used these principles to place the tibial component in 10–15° of internal rotation corresponding to knee mechanics driving the femur into internal rotation of approximately 20° on the tibia at full extension.

7.3.4   Patellofemoral Arthroplasty

Original designs for patellofemoral arthroplasty (PFA) resurfaced only the patella; however, the second-generation designs incorporated a trochlear component due to the persistence of knee pain after patella resurfacing. PFA is ideal for a patient with arthritis as a result of patellofemoral dysplasia without maltracking. Any medial or lateral joint line tenderness should be a strict contraindication to PFA with consideration made for other more extensive treatment options. The indications for PFA are listed in Table 7.3.

7.4   Controversies

7.4.1   Deficient ACL in Young Patients

7.4.1.1 Medial UKA
There has historically been controversy surrounding the extent to which an ACL deficiency is a contraindication to MUKA. In a cadaveric kinematic study, Suggs et al. [30] demonstrated a larger anterior translation of the tibia on the femur in ACL-deficient static-bearing MUKA. The authors speculated that this instability would create an environment in which further lateral and patellofemoral compartment wear would ensue. The mechanics of the Suggs study were tested by Argenson et al. [31] who found that when an ACL-deficient MUKA was in extension, the femur had a posterior contact position on the tibia. They also observed a paradoxical anterior translation of the femur on the tibia, which is also thought to play a role in accelerated wear of the polyethylene bearing.

Despite the above studies and their findings, some studies have suggested that good to equivocal results and survivorship could be expected in ACL-deficient knees [32–34]. One of the criteria for such outcomes was that the tibial component had to be positioned at <7° slope. These studies were not specifically focused on younger patients nor their expected increased activity level and demand on durability.

The ambiguity in whether or not to include ACL deficiency as a contraindication for UKA seems to swing from controversial to absolute in the younger population if the ACL instability is not addressed as well. In a recent study, Biswas et al. [7] offered ACL reconstruction at the time of their UKA in patients with ACL-deficient knees who were candidates for UKA. Results at a 2-year follow-up estimated a survival of 96.5 % at 10 years. Given the younger patient's expected higher activity level and life expectancy, unaddressed ACL deficiency as a contraindication seems consistent among the studies related to UKA in younger patients [3, 19, 25, 7, 15, 35].

Given the above data, we recommend an algorithm based on Weston-Simmons et al. [36]. This stems from understanding the pathologic process of medial compartment osteoarthritis (MCOA) and its etiology. If arthritis is the primary pathology, it will extend from an anterior to posterior direction leading to progressive ACL destruction. As this is a chronic process, by the time the ACL is damaged, the MCL and lateral compartment are affected, thus precluding the use of a UKA. If ACL deficiency is the primary pathology, the arthritic changes begin posteriorly as a result of

Fig 7.1 Algorithm for treatment of medial compartment OA with ACL tear

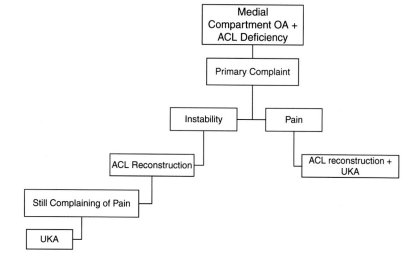

the posterior femoral subluxation in relation to the tibia. If a patient with the later pathologic process presents to clinic, the decision to treat both the ACL and MCOA in a single procedure is based on their primary complaint. If instability is the primary complaint, an ACL reconstruction is performed first. Should the primary complaint be pain, both an ACL reconstruction and UKA can be performed (see Fig. 7.1). With the use of this algorithm, the implant survival has been 93 %, with a patient satisfaction of 98 % [36].

7.4.1.2 Lateral UKA

LUKA in an ACL-deficient knee has been contraindicated in all patient populations due to the increased motion of the lateral compartment particularly in regard to anteroposterior translation. This has been shown to have a higher rate of failure in static and mobile-bearing prostheses in ACL-deficient knees [13]. There is a paucity of data with regard to LUKA with ACL repair at the time of surgery and thus no recommendations as to the potential use of such surgical management.

Regardless of the patient, ACL reconstruction at the time of UKA should be reserved for the surgeon well experienced in both UKA and ACL reconstructions. Although the literature has supported UKA in ACL-deficient knees if they lack clinical or intraoperative instability, ACL reconstruction in clinically ACL-deficient patients

who are candidates for UKA may also be an outcome supported surgical option.

7.4.2 Asymptomatic PFJ Arthritis

Typically PFJ arthritis has been a contraindication to UKA, especially in the young patient. Concerns for incomplete relief of pain or progressive arthritic change in the years postoperatively following the partial knee replacement have led to this contraindication. Recently the swing has been for the surgeon to use physical exam as a guide of inclusion for a patient with PFJ arthritis, namely, does the patient have anterior knee pain [25]. Symptomatic PFJ arthritis is thought to be a contraindication to surgery and not necessarily as dependent on radiographic findings.

7.4.3 Mobile Versus Static Bearing

The challenge with reviewing the literature addressing fixed versus mobile bearings is that some of the published research involves components with older designs and issues for which the manufacturer has made substantial corrections. For example, in a retrospective review, Emerson et al. [37] reported a 99 % survivorship for the Oxford (Biomet, Warsaw, IN) meniscal-bearing design and 93 % for the Robert Brigham fixed-bearing design (Johnson & Johnson Orthopaedics, Raynham, MA), based on component loosening and revision. Concerns with this study include the author's choice of compared implants occurred during two different time periods and therefore may not account for changes in the technology or advances in the surgeon's skill and experience. Contrast that finding to one earlier on in the development of the Oxford, which showed mobile-bearing revision to be twice that of fixed-bearing revisions. The most common reason for revision was for dislocated poly [13].

Keeping this in mind, there are arguments to be made for both bearing options, and as the current literature is reviewed, the difficulties of both types are heavily technique dependent.

7.4.3.1 Pros

Mobile

The concept behind mobile-bearing surfaces is the reduction of shear forces due to the fully congruent and unconstrained design, thus giving the implant reduced wear rates. Studies suggest that due to the congruent nature of mobile bearings as well as the lack of constraint, there is minimal wear and shear forces and thus decreased chance of loosening of the tibia baseplate. Twenty-year in vivo wear rates have been reported to be as low as 0.4 mm with a 0.02 mm/year wear rate [38].

Static

One of the earliest static-bearing designs was the Marmor prosthesis (Smith & Nephew, Memphis, TN). The tibial component was cemented on cancellous bone within the cortical rim as an inlay prosthesis resulting in high levels of subsidence and failure. Metal backing was introduced in the 1980s in order to evenly distribute the forces across a wider area. With the modularity that the metal-backed components provide, femoral component implantation became easier and also allowed for an isolated poly exchange should the patient require it. Static bearings also eliminated concerns for spin out of the bearing and dislocation of the poly insert.

7.4.3.2 Cons

Mobile

The most commonly cited issue with mobile-bearing designs is the worry for poly dislocation. This is seen in both medial and lateral UKA patients. Gunther et al. [39] saw an increased risk in lateral UKA when compared to MUKA in a series of fifty-three patients. There was a 10 % rate of bearing dislocation and a 21 % failure rate at 5 years postoperatively. Although techniques and implant design have improved dislocation, it still remains a concern that needs to be considered when choosing a mobile bearing. Some designs such as the LCS (low contact stress) component (DePuy, Warsaw, IN) use a dovetail track to lower the chances of poly dislocation [13]. A meta-analysis of the Oxford UKA showed a dislocation rate of 0.4 %, which has been considered acceptable [40]. The difficulty with bearing dislocation in UKA is that it often is due to poor positioning of the implants, and thus, a full revision may need to be done in order to prevent future dislocations.

Static

Despite the advantages, the metal-backed design brings some disadvantages as well. A dichotomy between thinner poly and larger tibial bone cut is created, whereas the surgeon must take multiple factors into consideration when deciding on an implant. Studies have shown that the greatest success for fixed-bearing devices has come from round-on-flat or slightly dished geometries [13]. Concerns for increased wear of the poly due to higher constraint in static bearing designs have also been published. Increased wear in the second decade of patients under 60 years of age with fixed-bearing (Miller–Galante) UKA has been noted and should be taken into consideration when potentially recommending these designs to younger, active patients [41].

7.4.3.3 Outcomes

Recent literature has shown that mobile-bearing UKA in patients under 60 years has a similar rate of failure as in those over 60 years of age, including a survival of 97 % at 10 years [42]. There have been several studies showing the long-term benefit of fixed- and mobile-bearing UKA designs. Berger et al. [20] recently reported results of a modular fixed-bearing, metal-backed tibial component. The authors noted that their thinnest polyethylene was 5.7 mm and was used in more than half of their patients. They showed a survival of 96 % at an average of 12-year follow-up (minimum 10-year follow-up) with 92 % of patients having excellent or good outcomes. The average age was 68 years (range 51–84). The authors emphasized their strict patient selection (Kozinn and Scott) and surgical technique as reasons for their success.

Similarly, Price et al. [43] reported a survival of 93 % at 15 years with 91 % of patients having good or excellent results with a mobile bearing. The authors argued that the decreased polyethylene contact stresses resulting from the mobile bearing's congruent design allowed them to implant polyethylene liners as thin as 3.5 mm with no change in clinical outcome or failure rate. The clinical relevance of the thin polyethylene liner is that it allows for a smaller tibial bone cut and increased preservation of native bone to allow for more options at the time of a revision.

In a recent study, a comparable 20-year survivorship rate was found between the two bearing types with slight differences observed between the United Kingdom, North America, and Europe [44]. This is also supported by a paper that looked at revision rates between the two bearing types at 15-year follow-up. The authors considered revision for any reason to be an end point and showed 12 of 77 (15 %) UKAs were revised (for aseptic loosening, dislocation, and arthritis progression) in the mobile-bearing group and 10 of 79 (12 %) in the fixed-bearing group (for wear and arthritis progression) [45].

There has only been one prospective, randomized controlled study comparing mobile and static bearing [46]. The authors compared the AMC mobile-bearing component (Alphanorm, Quierschied, Germany) with the Allegretto fixed-bearing component (Centerpulse, Baar, Switzerland). At a mean 5.7-year follow-up, there was no statistically significant difference between the groups with regard to revision rates or clinical outcome scores.

Radiographically, the number of overcorrections and the number of radiolucencies tend to be statistically higher in the mobile-bearing group (69 % vs. 24 %); however, this doesn't seem to make a difference in revision rates [41].

Kinematic analysis has shown that the mobile-bearing UKA has normal kinematics at 1 and 10 years. Static UKA kinematics are normal at 1 year, but at 10 years, the kinematic profile deteriorates to that of a TKA [44]. The mean Knee Society function and knee scores were comparable in a recent study comparing the two types of bearing surfaces at 15 years [41].

7.4.3.4 Summary

Regardless of the bearing type selected by the surgeon, advances in technology as well as surgeon comfort level in dealing with not only the primary procedure but each complication associated with its given bearing type need to be thoroughly considered. The complications of each bearing result typically from component malposition. We recommend either bearing type as long as the surgeon is comfortable with component implantation and understands the kinematics of each implant design.

7.5 Unicompartmental Knee Arthroplasty Outcomes

7.5.1 Medial UKA

Age has not been reported to be a predictor of poor outcomes. In fact, in a recent study by Thompson et al. [47], there was no significant difference in Knee Society Score (KSS) at 1 year; however, at 2 years there was a statistically significant difference in KSS with patients <60 years old scoring higher (Fig. 7.2).

The outcomes for MUKA in young patients have been reported before, and there seems to be differing opinion between the studies conducted in the United States and those in Europe with regard to survival. For example, the Swedish Knee Arthroplasty Registry found a 10-year survival rate of 83 % in patients <65 years of age who received a UKA for osteoarthritis. However, there

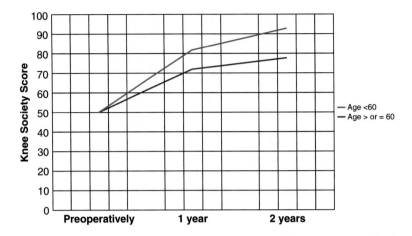

Fig 7.2 KSS scores in patients <60 and >60 years, 1 and 2 years post MUKA (Data from Thompson et al. [47]. *P*-value >0.05 at 1 year, which becomes significant (*p*-value 0.01) at 2 years postoperatively)

was no mention of patient selection or surgical experience, and the data included at least nine different prostheses [25]. Besides the lack of patient data, the registry data's lack of surgical experience data leaves the outcomes suspect as it has been reported that long-term results for unicompartmental arthroplasty are related to the number of surgeries performed by a given unit (study center) and reduce the failure of the UKA [48].

A recent study by Heyse et al. [49] studied lateral and medial UKA in patients <60 years old (average age at index operation – 53.7 (SD 5.8, range 30–60) years) with a mean follow-up of 10.8 years. The KSS was 94.3 (SD 7.8), and the function score was 94.9 (SD 6.8) with a 94.3 implant survival rate. Survivorship for the entire cohort was 93.5 % at 10 years (MUKA 94.1 % vs. lateral 91.8 %) and 86.3 % at 15 years (85.1 % medial vs. 91.7 % lateral). This seems to be consistent with other literature on MUKA in young patients (Table 7.4) [7, 49, 19, 50, 51, 25, 52].

7.5.2 Lateral UKA

The prevalence of lateral knee compartment osteoarthritis has been reported to be much lower than the other compartments which, by nature, leads to a lack of data regarding LUKA especially in younger patients [54]. It has been reported that MUKA is performed in a 10:1 ratio to LUKA [55]. Outcomes reported for LUKA however have been favorable. In one study,

authors looked at 29 LUKAs. At an average of 12.4-year follow-up (range of 3.1–15.6), all of their implants were functioning and no revisions. On average, they also saw the HSS knee scores increase from 60 to 93 postoperatively [27].

Smith et al. [28] saw a 98.7 % and 95.5 % survival of 100 lateral UKA patients at 2 and 5 years, respectively. The authors also saw AKSS (best 100, worst 0) and WOMAC (best 7, worst 35) scores improve after surgery. Median AKS function score increased from a preoperative score of 55–90 at 5 years. Median WOMAC function scores also improved from 22 preoperatively to 11 at 5 years.

Sah and Scott [56] published a series of 49 knees, using three different prostheses. They showed a survivorship of 100 % at 5.2-year follow-up. Studies with longer follow-up (10 years) have been published by Argenson et al. [57] and Lustig et al. [58] and report 92 % and 98 % prostheses survival, respectively.

Again, when compared to recently published data for all lateral UKA performed in England and Wales from the National Joint Registry [59], the results of Smith et al. present more favorably, which shows the discrepancy between outcomes in independent series, inventor studies, and registries [28].

7.5.3 PFA

There is a paucity of data for young patients undergoing PFA. The most recent review looked at 16 publications addressing PFA outcomes (total

Table 7.4 Summary of literature reporting results of MUKR in young patients

Study	Year	Age	ROM preoperatively (°)	ROM postoperatively (°)	Mean KSS preoperatively	Mean KSS postoperatively	Survival (years)	UCLA activity score at follow-up
Biswas et al. [7]	2014	49	120	124	49	95.1	96.5 % at 10 years (95 % confidence interval, 89.4 %–98.8 %)	7.5
Dalury et al. [53]	2013	46–59				Significant increase postoperatively	94.1 % at 6 years (95 % CI, 78.3–98.5)	
Heyse et al. [49][a]	2012	53.7			50.1	94.3	93.5 % at 10 years, 91.3 % at 12 years, and 86.3 % at 15 years (MUKA was 94.1 % at 10 years, 91.2 % at 12 years, and 85.1 % at 15 years) (91.8 % at 10 and 15 years for LUKA)	
Felts et al. [19]	2010	54.7	110	132	50	94	94 % at 12 years (95 % CI, 0.87–0.96)	6.8
Parratte et al. [50]	2009	46	110	132	54	97	80.6 % at 12 years and 70 % at 16 years	
Cartier et al. [51]	2007	53		116		94.02	94 % at 10 years, 92 % at 11 years, and 88 % at 12 years	
Price et al. [25]	2005	<60	109	116			91 % at 10 years (95 % CI 12.4)	
Schai et al. [52][a]	1998	52	117	124	52	93		

[a]Included LUKAs

of 773 patients and 912 knees) with an average age of 55.9 years (range 19–90 years) and a mean follow-up of 5.7 years (range 0.16–24 years). The outcomes showed an average of 88 % improved function and pain relief (range 42–96 %) [60].

One study specifically looked at patients under the age of 55 undergoing PFA. The authors made specific mention of a unique prerequisite with regard to the patient's mental state and more specifically that it is stable. They looked at 110 patients and found a less predictable benefit to PFA when compared with MUKA [61].

Overall, PFA has been somewhat controversial and unpredictable which is likely related to most of the early studies using first-generation implants [60]. Patient selection is also of utmost importance when considering PFA.

7.6   Return to Activity

It comes to no surprise that young patients seek care for joint pain that limits their activity level and quality of life. The question most difficult to address is whether these patients will or should be able to return to impact activities or will they be forever limited in their activities post-UKA.

For the patients who are inactive in regard to sport, there is very little evidence to prove that they will become actively involved in a new activity postoperatively. What the literature does show is that postoperatively, there will be a return to activity rate of 94.8 % at the same frequency at which the patient participated preoperatively [62]. While the participation remains high in the postoperative period, there are some things to keep in mind.

The number of patients who perform 60 min of activity at a time has been shown to significantly decrease. What will also change is the type of activities. In the younger patients (<66 years old), three of the top five sport activities (tennis, downhill skiing, hiking) showed a significant decrease of participation of 84.5, 51.9, and 28.0 %, respectively, in the postoperative period [62]. The other two activities, cycling and swimming, showed no significant decrease in participation.

Given the above information, it is important to also note that patients who undergo UKA will have a significantly higher health-related quality of life as measured by the SF-36 questionnaire than people in the same demographic who have not undergone UKA [62].

7.6.1   Recommendations

We recommend patients receive a rapid therapy protocol with range of motion and mobilization beginning as quickly as possible in the postoperative period. After the initial postoperative visit, patients can return to work and driving if they meet the following criteria:

1. Are not taking any narcotic pain medication
2. Are not needing an assistive device to ambulate
3. Have complete voluntary control of their operative extremity
4. Have practiced in a low-stakes environment (e.g., empty parking lot)

We recommend the surgeon counsel their patients with regard to high-impact activities and the potential of increased wear and loosening rates which could ultimately lead to early implant failure and need for revision surgery. Patients should be symptom- and pain-free during their chosen activities and should have undergone a muscular rehab protocol focused on strengthening the quadriceps and hamstring muscles and overall conditioning of the extremity prior to participation in sport activities.

It should be recommended that patients participate in activities that are low and mid-impact exercises such as swimming, cycling, hiking, weight training, golf, and skiing (excluding moguls and jumps).

7.7   Special Circumstances

7.7.1   Isolated Cartilage Lesion

7.7.1.1 Focal Femoral Condyle Resurfacing

Indications
There remains a dilemma when a patient presents with an isolated, full-thickness, one-sided

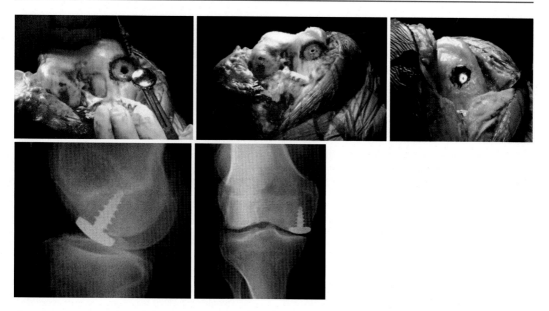

Fig. 7.3 HemiCAP procedure (Courtesy of Dr. Myles Coolican)

cartilage lesion. Results have been poor in middle-aged patients (40–60 years old) when they are treated with procedures amenable to a younger population (micro fracture, osteochondral grafting, and chondrocyte implantation) [63]. There is a paucity of data with regard to long-term outcomes; however, the criteria for inclusion of focal femoral condyle resurfacing (FFCR) are as follows:

- BMI <35
- One-sided defect (no kissing lesions)
- Diameter <20 mm
- Osteoarthritis (no inflammatory arthritis)
- No ligamentous instability
- Varus/valgus malalignment <7°

Postoperative Course
Standardized rehab is focused on range of motion followed by strengthening. The primary implant stability allows for rapid recovery and a symptom-based rehab progression protocol and weight bearing once postoperative pain and swelling has subsided [63] (Fig. 7.3).

Outcomes
Given the debilitating nature of a full-thickness cartilage lesion in an otherwise healthy knee, it comes to no surprise that satisfactory outcomes

result from FFCR. In a recent study, there was a significant increase in the HSS score with an average of 45 % increase in knee scores and 48 % in function scores from the pre- to postoperative period [63]. Another study looked at Knee Injury and Osteoarthritis Outcome Score (KOOS) scores at 5 years following FFCR and compared it to normative data for the same age demographic. All KOOS scores increased postoperatively and were significantly better for all components of the KOOS scores in females with the exception of the Sports and Recreation and Quality of Life components. When compared to normal males, the scores were inferior across the board [64]. Given the right pathology, FFCR can provide a good outcome while potentially buying time to more invasive reconstructive (UKA/TKA) procedures.

7.7.1.2 Patellofemoral Inlay Resurfacing

Indications
Patellofemoral arthritis is common in the younger, active population with high expectations postoperatively to return to a high level of function. Thorough history and physical with appropriate studies should allow the physician to determine which patient is a candidate for

patellofemoral inlay resurfacing (PFIR). Indications have classically included disabling patellofemoral OA (grades III–IV according to the Kellgren–Lawrence scale) or chondrosis (grades III–IV according to Outerbridge) that has been refractory to conservative treatment and/or prior surgery without any of the following [65]:

- Concomitant tibiofemoral OA creating pain during activities of daily living
- Systemic inflammatory arthropathy
- Chondrocalcinosis
- Chronic regional pain syndrome
- Fixed loss of knee range of motion

Postoperative Course
After isolated PFIR, weight bearing is limited for 2 weeks. Full range of motion can be allowed immediately; however, if there is another procedure performed concomitantly with PFIR, this may limit the ROM and weight-bearing protocol postoperatively.

Outcomes
Given the high demand that PFIR patients put on their knees, a majority (58 %) of them participate in athletics despite needing surgery [65]. Studies have shown that even if there is another procedure performed at the time of the PFIR (i.e., medial patellofemoral ligament reconstruction), patients will see an increase in their IKDC, WOMAC, visual analogue scale for pain (VAS) scores, as well as an increase in the postsurgical participation in athletics [65].

7.7.2 Bicompartmental Arthroplasty

Bicompartmental knee arthroplasty is defined as the simultaneous arthroplasty of either the medial or lateral compartment in addition to the PFJ. There are limited studies with regard to bicompartmental arthroplasty and outcomes. One study by Palumbo et al. [66] showed a 14 % revision rate for pain, and 39 % of patients had poor outcomes. The prosthesis used in the study is no longer used at the investigating institution.

Another study by Morrison et al. [67] showed a 14 % revision rate and a 28 % complication rate.

We recommend bicompartmental arthroplasty be performed only by those surgeons with high volume of knee arthroplasty as the procedure is very technique dependent and the potential complications are numerous in these cases.

7.7.3 Conversion to TKA

Most commonly cited reasons for UKA failure include bearing wear, loosening, and progression of DJD in the adjacent compartments. Studies have pointed to the progression of arthritis in the other compartments and component loosening as the highest reasons for UKA revision surgery. One study revealed 51 % of revision surgeries were due to adjacent DJD, while another study favored loosening (43 %) as the most common cause. Both articles agreed that the two most common reasons for revision surgery of a UKA are progression of arthritis and component loosening [13]. A recent study using data in the Finnish Arthroplasty Registry found that in younger patients (<or=65 years of age), there was a 1.5-fold increased risk of revision compared to older patients [2]. What still remains a challenge when interpreting data on UKA is the difference in findings between data registries and smaller studies with registries typically reporting poorer outcomes.

A recent study by Craik et al. [68] showed that the risk of early revision surgery was greater in patients with MUKA compared with primary TKA. An interesting point was made regarding the loss of bone stock and variation of functional scores with UKAs needing revision surgery. The authors stated that poor pre-revision function dictated post-revision function regardless of the need for additional intraoperative measures to make up for loss of bone stock. They concluded that in the case where a patient's function was deteriorating after primary UKA, expedition of revision surgery might be warranted to improve function after revision surgery. This is backed by Pearse's study, which stated that UKA to TKA revisions do worse than primary TKA and have a fourfold increase in revision rates thereafter.

Fig. 7.4 AP (**a**) and lateral (**b**) preoperative x-rays of a failed MUKA

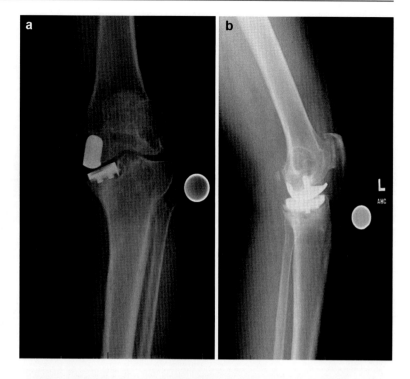

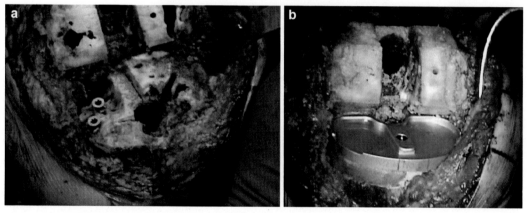

Fig. 7.5 Intraoperative management of medial bone defects with screws (**a**) and medial wedge (**b**)

However, if a UKA in a young patient is going to fail because of wear, it has been discussed that a TKA in that same patient would fail for the same reason [19, 69]. Furthermore, it has been proposed that UKA to TKA may be more straightforward than TKA to revision TKA [4].

In the instances where a UKA to TKA revision was required, the outcomes have been good. There have been few studies of UKA revisions; however, the data is promising. Levine et al. [70] showed good results at an average follow-up of 45 months for UKA's revised to TKA at an average of 62 months. No structural allografts were needed, and they mentioned that their revisions were comparable to primary TKA. A similar study of 73 revisions at an average of 58 months had small bone defects and a total of 20 requiring bone graft of wedges. They reported 80 % excellent or good results at an average of 56-month follow-up [71]. Figures 7.4, 7.5, and 7.6 illustrate reconstruction of failed MUKA converted to TKA with augments for significant bone loss.

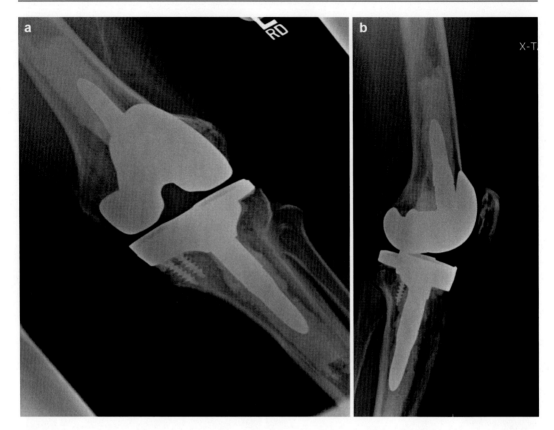

Fig. 7.6 AP (**a**) and lateral (**b**) postoperative radiographs showing screw and wedge augments as well as short cemented stems

7.8   Surgical Pearls

Technical errors in UKA can lead to early revision procedures as can poor patient selection. The following are considerations when undertaking these procedures to increase the likelihood of good clinical outcomes.

7.8.1   Medial UKA

- Don't let minimal exposure dictate poor implant position.
- ACL competence is important.
- Volume will improve outcomes.
- Do not overcorrect varus/valgus deformities.

7.8.2   Lateral UKA

- Tibia component must be internally rotated for appropriate tracking.
- ACL must be competent.
  - Do not overcorrect varus/valgus deformities.

7.8.3   PFA

- Must be very selective about patients, good candidates rare.
- Prominent femoral components will fail.
- Skin incision should be conducive to potentiate future TKA incision.

7.8.4 FFCR

Given that a focal chondral lesion may result from trauma, it is imperative that the surgeon rule out other concomitant lesions or be willing to address them at the time of surgery. We recommend a diagnostic arthroscopy prior to proceeding with FFCR to look for other pathology and to ensure the patient is a candidate for the procedure. More specifically, addressing any meniscal tear is essential to satisfaction and prosthetic life. Failure to treat meniscal pathology has been shown to increase contact pressure 78 % during dynamic range of motion [72].

7.8.5 PFIR

As is the case with FFCR, it is imperative that the surgeon considers concomitant pathologies, which may contribute to the symptoms of a patient presenting with an isolated PFJ lesion. The surgeon should be comfortable with tibial tubercle transfers, distal femoral osteotomies, high tibial osteotomies, lateral retinacular releases, and medial patellofemoral ligament reconstruction as all have been shown to be potentially needed at the time of PFIR [65].

References

1. Palumbo BT, Scott RD. Diagnosis and indications for treatment of unicompartmental arthritis. Clin Sports Med. 2014;33(02785919):11–21.
2. Koskinen E, Paavolainen P, Eskelinen A, Pulkkinen P, Remes V. Unicondylar knee replacement for primary osteoarthritis: a prospective follow-up study of 1,819 patients from the Finnish Arthroplasty Register. Acta Orthop. 2007;78:128–35.
3. W-Dahl A, Robertsson O, Lidgren L, Miller L, Davidson D, Graves S. Unicompartmental knee arthroplasty in patients aged less than 65: combined data from the Australian and Swedish Knee Registries. Acta Orthop [En ligne]. 2010;81:90–4. Disponible: http://www.scopus.com/inward/record.url?eid=2-s2.0-77950473777&partnerID=40&md5=6ecfab0a58ab4761ac1cb85747efee61.
4. Pearse AJ, Hooper GJ, Rothwell A, Frampton C. Survival and functional outcome after revision of a unicompartmental to a total knee replacement: the New Zealand National Joint Registry. J Bone Joint Surg Br. 2010;92(4):508–12.
5. Baker PN, Petheram T, Avery PJ, Gregg PJ, Deehan DJ. Revision for unexplained pain following unicompartmental and total knee replacement. J Bone Joint Surg Am. 2012;94:e126.
6. Laurencin CT, Zelicof SB, Scott RD, Ewald FC. Unicompartmental versus total knee arthroplasty in the same patient. A comparative study. Clin Orthop Relat Res. 1991;273:151–6.
7. Biswas D, Van Thiel GS, Wetters NG, Pack BJ, Berger RA, Della Valle CJ. Medial unicompartmental knee arthroplasty in patients less than 55 years old: minimum of two years of follow-up. J Arthroplasty [En ligne]. Elsevier Inc.; 2014;29(1):101–5. Disponible: http://dx.doi.org/10.1016/j.arth.2013.04.046.
8. Saccomanni B. Unicompartmental knee arthroplasty: a review of literature. Clin Rheumatol. 2010;29(4):339–46.
9. [En ligne]. Swedish Knee Arthroplasty Register Annual Report. 2014 [cité le 23 mai 2015]. Disponible: http://myknee.se/pdf/SKAR2014_Eng_1.1.pdf.
10. Australian Orthopaedic Association National Joint Replacement Registry. Annual Report [En ligne]. Adelaide: AOA. 2014. Disponible: https://aoanjrr.dmac.adelaide.edu.au/documents/10180/172286/Annual. Report 2014.
11. Wishart N, Beaumont R, Young E, Mccormack V, Swanson M. National Joint Registry for England, Wales and Northern Ireland: 11th Annual Report [En ligne]. 2014. Disponible: http://www.njrcentre.org.uk/njrcentre/Portals/0/Documents/England/Reports/11th_annual_report/NJR. 11th Annual Report 2014.pdf.
12. Rothwell A, Larmer P, Hobbs T, Rothwell A. The New Zealand Joint Registry Annual Report Editorial Committee. 2014. Disponible: http://www.nzoa.org.nz/system/files/NZJR2014Report.pdf.
13. Borus T, Thornhill T. Unicompartmental knee arthroplasty. J Am Acad Orthop Surg. 2008;16:9–18.
14. Journal T, Vol A, Schai A, Scott D. Unicompartmental knee arthroplasty in middle – aged patients a 2- to 6-year follow-up evaluation. J Anthroplasty. 1998;13(4):365–72.
15. Deshmukh RV, Scott RD. Unicompartmental knee arthroplasty for younger patients: an alternative view. Clin Orthop Relat Res. 2002;(404):108–12.
16. Mariani EM, Bourne MH, Jackson RT, Jackson ST, Jones P. Recalled-early failure of unicompartmental knee arthroplasty. J Arthroplasty. 2007;22(6):81–4.
17. Fehring TK, Odum SM, Masonis JL, Springer BD. Early failures in unicondylar arthroplasty. Orthopedics. 2010;33:11.
18. Kozinn SC, Scott R. Unicondylar knee arthroplasty. J Bone Joint Surg Am. 1989;71(I):145–50.

19. Felts E, Parratte S, Pauly V, Aubaniac J-M, Argenson J-N. Function and quality of life following medial unicompartmental knee arthroplasty in patients 60 years of age or younger. Orthop Traumatol Surg Res [En ligne]. 2010;96(8):861–7. Disponible: http://www.sciencedirect.com/science/article/pii/S1877056810002057.

20. Berger RA, Meneghini RM, Jacobs JJ, Sheinkop MB, Della Valle CJ, Rosenberg AG, et al. Results of unicompartmental knee arthroplasty at a minimum of ten years of follow-up. J Bone Joint Surg Am [En ligne]. The Journal of Bone and Joint Surgery, Inc. 2005 [cité le 28 févr 2015];87(5):999–1006. Disponible: http://jbjs.org/content/87/5/999.abstract.

21. Murray DW, Pandit H, Weston-Simons JS, Jenkins C, Gill HS, Lombardia V, et al. Does body mass index affect the outcome of unicompartmental knee replacement? Knee [En ligne]. 2012;20(6):461–5. Disponible: http://www.ncbi.nlm.nih.gov/pubmed/23110877.

22. Broughton NS, Newman JH, Baily RA. Unicompartmental replacement and high tibial osteotomy for osteoarthritis of the knee. A comparative study after 5–10 years' follow-up. J Bone Joint Surg Br. 1986;68:447–52.

23. Psychoyios V, Crawford RW, O'Connor JJ, Murray DW. Wear of congruent meniscal bearings in unicompartmental knee arthroplasty: a retrieval study of 16 specimens. J Bone Joint Surg Br. 1998;80:976–82.

24. Munk B, Frøkjaer J. A 10-year follow-up of unicompartmental arthrosis treated with the Marmor method. Ugeskr Laeger. 1994;156:4029–31.

25. Price AJ, Dodd CAF, Svard UGC, Murray DW. Oxford medial unicompartmental knee arthroplasty in patients younger and older than 60 years of age. J Bone Jt Surg Br [En ligne]. 2005;87:1488–92. Disponible: C:\Users\Public\Documents\10 PubMed Literatur\2005\JBJS-B\Price2005b - Oxford medial UKA in patients younger and older than 60 years.pdf.

26. Niinimäki TT, Murray DW, Partanen J, Pajala A, Leppilahti JI. Unicompartmental knee arthroplasties implanted for osteoarthritis with partial loss of joint space have high re-operation rates. Knee. 2011;18:432–5.

27. Pennington DW, Swienckowski JJ, Lutes WB, Drake GN. Lateral unicompartmental knee arthroplasty: survivorship and technical considerations at an average follow-up of 12.4 years. J Arthroplasty [En ligne]. 2006 [cité le 24 janv 2015];21(1):13–7. Disponible: http://www.sciencedirect.com/science/article/pii/S0883540305001336.

28. Smith JRA, Robinson JR, Porteous AJ, Murray JRD, Hassaballa MA, Artz N, et al. The knee fixed bearing lateral unicompartmental knee arthroplasty — short to mid-term survivorship and knee scores for 101 prostheses. Knee [En ligne]. Elsevier B.V.; 2014;21(4):843–7. Disponible: http://dx.doi.org/10.1016/j.knee.2014.04.003.

29. Lonner JH. Patellofemoral arthroplasty. J Am Acad Orthop Surg. 2007;15(8):495–506.

30. Suggs JF, Li G, Park SE, Steffensmeier S, Rubash HE, Freiberg AA. Function of the anterior cruciate ligament after unicompartmental knee arthroplasty: an in vitro robotic study. J Arthroplasty. 2004;19:224–9.

31. Argenson J-NA, Komistek RD, Aubaniac J-M, Dennis DA, Northcut EJ, Anderson DT, et al. In vivo determination of knee kinematics for subjects implanted with a unicompartmental arthroplasty. J Arthroplasty. 2002;17:1049–54.

32. Christensen NO. Unicompartmental prosthesis for gonarthrosis. A nine-year series of 575 knees from a Swedish hospital. Clin Orthop Relat Res. 1991;165–9.

33. Hernigou P, Deschamps G. Posterior slope of the tibial implant and the outcome of unicompartmental knee arthroplasty. J Bone Joint Surg Am. 2004;86-A:506–11.

34. Cartier P, Sanouiller JL, Grelsamer RP. Unicompartmental knee arthroplasty surgery. 10-year minimum follow-up period. J Arthroplasty. 1996;11(7):782–8.

35. Pennington DW, Swienckowski JJ, Lutes WB, Drake GN, Pennington DW. Unicompartmental knee arthroplasty in patients sixty years of age or younger. J Bone Joint Surg Am. 2003;85-A:1968–73.

36. Weston-Simons JS, Pandit H, Jenkins C, Jackson WFM, Price AJ, Gill HS, et al. Outcome of combined unicompartmental knee replacement and combined or sequential anterior cruciate ligament reconstruction: a study of 52 cases with mean follow-up of five years. J Bone Joint Surg Br. 2012;94:1216–20. Disponible: http://dx.doi.org/10.1302/0301-620X.94B9.28881.

37. Emerson RH, Hansborough T, Reitman RD, Rosenfeldt W, Higgins LL. Comparison of a mobile with a fixed-bearing unicompartmental knee implant. Clin Orthop Relat Res. 2002;62–70.

38. Kendrick BJL, Longino D, Pandit H, Svard U, Gill HS, Dodd CAF, et al. Polyethylene wear in Oxford unicompartmental knee replacement: a retrieval study of 47 bearings. J Bone Joint Surg Br. 2010;92(3):367–73.

39. Gunther TV, Murray DW, Miller R, Wallace DA, Carr AJ, O'Connor JJ, et al. Lateral unicompartmental arthroplasty with the Oxford meniscal knee. Knee [En ligne]. Elsevier; 1996 [cité le 28 févr 2015];3(1–2):33–9. Disponible: http://www.thekneejournal.com/article/0968016096002086/fulltext.

40. Kim S-J, Postigo R, Koo S, Kim JH. Causes of revision following Oxford phase 3 unicompartmental knee arthroplasty. Knee Surg Sport Traumatol Arthrosc [En ligne]. 2013;22(8):1895–901. Disponible: http://link.springer.com/10.1007/s00167-013-2644-3.

41. Argenson J-NA, Blanc G, Aubaniac J-M, Parratte S. Modern unicompartmental knee arthroplasty with cement: a concise follow-up, at a mean of twenty years, of a previous report. J Bone Joint Surg Am [En ligne]. 2013;95:905–9. Disponible: http://jbjs.org/article.aspx?articleid=1686214.

42. Pandit H, Jenkins C, Gill HS, Smith G, Price AJ, Dodd CA, Murray DW, et al. Unnecessary contraindications for mobile-bearing unicompartmental knee replacement. J Bone Joint Surg Br. 2011;93:622–8.

43. Price AJ, Orth F, Waite JC, Svard U. Long-term clinical results of the medial Oxford unicompartmental knee arthroplasty. Clin Orthop Relat Res. 2005;171–80.

44. Whittaker JP, Naudie DDR, McAuley JP, McCalden RW, MacDonald SJ, Bourne RB. Does bearing design

influence midterm survivorship of unicompartmental arthroplasty? Dans: Clin Orthop Relat Res. 2010; 468(1):73–81.

45. Parratte S, Pauly V, Aubaniac JM, Argenson JNA. No long-term difference between fixed and mobile medial unicompartmental arthroplasty. Dans: Clin Orthop Relat Res. 2012;470(1):61–8.

46. Confalonieri N, Manzotti A, Pullen C. Comparison of a mobile with a fixed tibial bearing unicompartimental knee prosthesis: a prospective randomized trial using a dedicated outcome score. Knee. 2004;11:357–62.

47. Thompson SAJ, Liabaud B, Nellans KW, Geller JA. Factors associated with poor outcomes following unicompartmental knee arthroplasty: redefining the "classic" indications for surgery. J Arthroplasty [En ligne]. Elsevier Inc.; 2013;28(9):1561–4. Disponible: http://www.sciencedirect.com/science/article/pii/S0883540313002052.

48. Robertsson O, Knutson K, Lewold S, Lidgren L. The routine of surgical management reduces failure after unicompartmental knee arthroplasty. J Bone Joint Surg Br. 2001;83(1):45–9.

49. Heyse TJ, Khefacha A, Peersman G, Cartier P. Survivorship of UKA in the middle-aged. Knee [En ligne]. Elsevier; 2012 [cité le 28 févr 2015];19(5):585–91. Disponible: http://www.thekneejournal.com/article/S0968016011001645/fulltext.

50. Parratte S, Argenson JN, Pearce O, Pauly V, Auquier P, Aubaniac JM. Medial unicompartmental knee replacement in the under-50s. J Bone Joint Surg Br. 2009; 91(3):351–6.

51. Cartier P, Khefacha A, Sanouiller J-L, Frederick K. Unicondylar knee arthroplasty in middle-aged patients: a minimum 5-year follow-up. Orthopedics. 2007;30:62–5.

52. Schai PA, Suh JT, Thornhill TS, Scott RD. Unicompartmental knee arthroplasty in middle-aged patients: a 2- to 6-year follow-up evaluation. J Arthroplasty. 1998;13:365–72.

53. Dalury D, Kelley TC, Adams MJ. Medial UKA: favorable mid-term results in middle-aged patients. J Knee Surg. 2013;26(2):133–7.

54. McAlindon TE, Snow S, Cooper C, Dieppe PA. Radiographic patterns of osteoarthritis of the knee joint in the community: the importance of the patellofemoral joint. Ann Rheum Dis [En ligne]. 1992 [cité le 28 févr 2015];51(7):844–9. Disponible: http://ard.bmj.com/cgi/content/long/51/7/844.

55. Scott RD. Lateral unicompartmental replacement: a road less traveled. Orthopedics. 2005;28:983–4.

56. Sah AP, Scott RD. Lateral unicompartmental knee arthroplasty through a medial approach. Study with an average five-year follow-up. J Bone Joint Surg Am [En ligne]. The Journal of Bone and Joint Surgery, Inc.; 2007 [cité le 27 févr 2015];89(9):1948–54. Disponible: http://jbjs.org/content/89/9/1948.abstract.

57. Argenson JNA, Parratte S, Bertani A, Flecher X, Aubaniac JM. Long-term results with a lateral unicondylar replacement. Dans: Clinical Orthopaedics and Related Research. 2008;466(11):2686–93.

58. Lustig S, Elguindy A, Servien E, Fary C, Munini E, Demey G, et al. 5- to 16-year follow-up of 54 consecutive lateral unicondylar knee arthroplasties with a fixed-all polyethylene bearing. J Arthroplasty [En ligne]. Elsevier Inc.; 2011 [cité le 28 févr 2015];26(8):1318–25. Disponible: http://www.arthroplastyjournal.org/article/S0883540311000398/fulltext.

59. Baker PN, Jameson SS, Deehan DJ, Gregg PJ, Porter M, Tucker K. Mid-term equivalent survival of medial and lateral unicondylar knee replacement: an analysis of data from a National Joint Registry. J Bone Joint Surg Br [En ligne]. 2012;94(12):1641–8. Disponible: http://www.ncbi.nlm.nih.gov/pubmed/23188905.

60. Leadbetter WB. Patellofemoral arthroplasty in the treatment of patellofemoral arthritis: rationale and outcomes in younger patients. Orthop Clin North Am. 2008;39:363–80.

61. Newman JH. Patellofemoral arthritis and its management with isolated patellofemoral replacement: a personal experience. Orthopedics. 2007;30:58–61.

62. Naal FD, Fischer M, Preuss A, Goldhahn J, von Knoch F, Preiss S, et al. Return to sports and recreational activity after unicompartmental knee arthroplasty. Am J Sports Med. 2007;35(10):1688–95.

63. Bollars P, Bosquet M, Vandekerckhove B, Hardeman F, Bellemans J. Prosthetic inlay resurfacing for the treatment of focal, full thickness cartilage defects of the femoral condyle: a bridge between biologics and conventional arthroplasty. Knee Surg Sport Traumatol Arthrosc. 2012;20(9):1753–9.

64. Becher C, Kalbe C, Thermann H, Paessler HH, Laprell H, Kaiser T, et al. Minimum 5-year results of focal articular prosthetic resurfacing for the treatment of full-thickness articular cartilage defects in the knee. Arch Orthop Trauma Surg. 2011;131(8):1135–43.

65. Imhoff AB, Feucht MJ, Meidinger G, Schöttle PB, Cotic M. Prospective evaluation of anatomic patellofemoral inlay resurfacing: clinical, radiographic, and sports-related results after 24 months. Knee Surg, Sport Traumatol Arthrosc [En ligne]. 2013;23(5):1299–307. Disponible: http://link.springer.com/10.1007/s00167-013-2786-3.

66. Palumbo BT, Henderson ER, Edwards PK, Burris RB, Gutiérrez S, Raterman SJ. Initial experience of the journey-deuce bicompartmental knee prosthesis: a review of 36 cases. J Arthroplasty [En ligne]. Elsevier Inc.; 2011;26(Suppl 6):40–5. Disponible: http://dx.doi.org/10.1016/j.arth.2011.03.026.

67. Morrison TA, Nyce JD, Macaulay WB, Geller JA. Early adverse results with bicompartmental knee arthroplasty: a prospective cohort comparison to total knee arthroplasty. J Arthroplasty. 2011;26 Suppl 6:35–9.

68. Craik JD, El Shafie SA, Singh VK, Twyman RS. Revision of unicompartmental knee arthroplasty versus primary total knee arthroplasty. J Arthroplasty [En ligne]. Elsevier; 2014 [cité le 28 févr 2015];30(4):592–4. Disponible: http://www.arthroplastyjournal.org/article/S0883540314008274/fulltext

69. Argenson J-NA, Parratte S. The unicompartmental knee: design and technical considerations in minimizing wear. Clin Orthop Relat Res. 2006;452:137–42.

70. Levine WN, Ozuna RM, Scott RD, Thornhill TS. Conversion of failed modern unicompartmental arthroplasty to total knee arthroplasty. J Arthroplasty. 1996;11(7):797–801.

71. Chakrabarty G, Newman JH, Ackroyd CE. Revision of unicompartmental arthroplasty of the knee: clinical and technical considerations. J Arthroplasty. 1998;13(2):191–6.

72. Becher C, Huber R, Thermann H, Tibesku CO, von Skrbensky G. Tibiofemoral contact mechanics with a femoral resurfacing prosthesis and a non-functional meniscus. Clin Biomech. 2009;24(8):648–54.

Total Knee Arthroplasty for the Young, Active Patient with Osteoarthritis

8

Tiffany N. Castillo and James I. Huddleston

Contents

T.N. Castillo, MD • J.I. Huddleston, MD (✉)
Department of Orthopaedic Surgery,
Stanford University Medical Center,
Stanford, CA, USA
e-mail: tiffanyc@stanford.edu;
jhuddleston@stanford.edu

8.1 Introduction

The demographic profile and expectations of patients with tricompartmental knee osteoarthritis who are seeking surgical treatment have shifted over the past several decades. Patients today tend to be younger and more active and seek rapid recovery, while also demand return to high-performance activities and optimal durability characteristics of their total knee components. Consequently, it is critical that surgeons understand the performance and survivability of total knee arthroplasty (TKA) in the young patient and appropriately counsel patients about postoperative expectations for pain relief, function, and durability.

8.2 Epidemiology

In 2013, the 1st Annual Report of the American Joint Replacement Registry revealed that the majority (62 %) of reported cases were knee procedures and the average age for all knee procedures (66.7 years) was less than that for hip procedures (67.6 years, Fig. 8.1).

The 2014 Australian Joint Registry Annual Report also supports this trend, with there being an increase in the number of total knee replacements in patients aged 55–64 years, while there is a relative status quo versus decrease in prevalence among all other age groups (Fig. 8.2).

© ISAKOS 2016

D.A. Parker (ed.), *Management of Knee Osteoarthritis in the Younger, Active Patient:*
An Evidence-Based Practical Guide for Clinicians, DOI 10.1007/978-3-662-48530-9_8

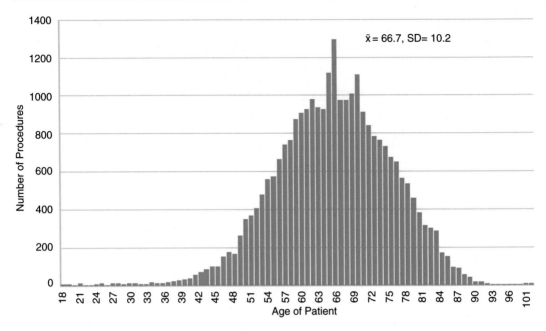

Fig. 8.1 Age distribution of all knee procedures ($N=27{,}158$) in the United States in 2013. The mean age (66.7 years) reflects the decreasing age at which knee procedures are being performed (2013 1st Annual Report of the American Joint Replacement Registry)

Fig. 8.2 Primary total knee replacement by age (Orthopaedic Association National Joint Replacement Registry. Annual Report. Adelaide: AOA, 2014)

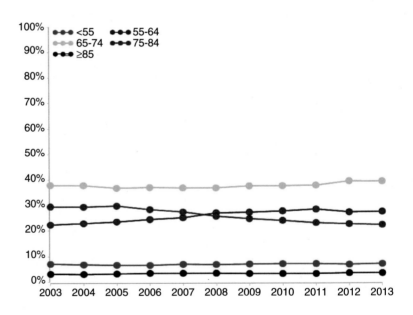

8.3   Survivorship

With the decreasing mean age of patients receiving total knee arthroplasties, a discussion about the durability of the components and the likelihood of the need for revision becomes paramount.

In the 2014 Australian Joint Registry Annual Report [1], the cumulative incidence of revision after primary total knee arthroplasty was in the order of 2 % for aseptic loosening and 1 % for infection. When analyzing the rates of revision by age, patients less than 55 made up the highest

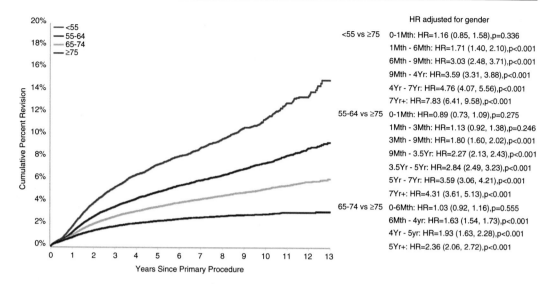

Fig. 8.3 Cumulative percent revision of primary total knee replacement for osteoarthritis by age (Orthopaedic Association National Joint Replacement Registry. Annual Report. Adelaide: AOA, 2014)

cumulative percent revision for primary total knee arthroplasty in every year after the primary procedure when compared to groups aged 55–64, 65–74, and greater than 75 years (Fig. 8.3).

When controlling for gender, the hazard ratio was greatest (7.83) when comparing cumulative percent revision for those less than 55 years to those greater than 75 years at 7+ years post primary total knee arthroplasty.

In the United States, the reasons for revision knee arthroplasty have changed over the last couple of decades. In the early 2000s, Sharkey et al. showed that the leading reasons for revision were polyethylene wear (25 %), loosening (24 %), instability (21 %), infection (18 %), arthrofibrosis (15 %), and malalignment (12 %) [2]. When looking at the time to revision, the majority (56 %) of these were early failures (less than 2 years after primary total knee arthroplasty), and among these early failures, infection was the leading cause for revision. Whereas in the late failure (greater than 2 years postprimary TKA), the leading causes for revision were polyethylene wear, loosening, and instability.

In 2010, a nationwide inpatient sample of over 60,000 patients from 2005 to 2006 revealed that infection was the leading reason for revision at 25 %, followed by mechanical loosening (16 %),

implant failure (10 %), wear and lysis (8 %), dislocation (7 %), and fracture (1.5 %) [3]. In 2014, Sharkey et al. published a follow-up study comparing reasons for revision knee arthroplasty in 2012 to those in 2002, which also demonstrated that while the overall most common reason for revision was loosening (40 %), infection (28 %) was by far the most common reason for early revisions [4]. A multicenter study by Schroer et al. in 2013 found instability to be the most common reason (25.2 %) for early (<2 years since primary TKA) revision TKA, followed by infection (22.8 %) [5]. A single-center study by Le et al. in 2014 also found a similar trend with instability (26 %) and infection (24 %) as the leading reasons for early revision TKA [6].

The reasons for infection and loosening resulting in higher rates of early failure of TKA are not entirely understood and remain an ongoing area of research. Bozic et al. recently reviewed a sample of >117,000 Medicare patients from 1998 to 2010 who had revision TKA within 12 months of their index operations and found that there were a number of associated medical comorbidities and modifiable risk factors: chronic obstructive pulmonary disease, depression, alcohol and drug abuse, renal disease, and obesity [7]. Although this study was done in an older cohort, it is reasonable to infer that these same risk factors should be identified and addressed in counseling younger patients considering TKA about potential postoperative complications.

8.4   Fixation

Since the durability and survivability of components are paramount in the young, active patient who undergoes TKA, many studies have attempted to analyze whether there is an optimal fixation modality, bearing mobility, bearing material, and level of constraint for such a patient population.

Although the original cementless TKA designs had limited survivorship due to metal-backed patellae, patch porous coating, and screw holes, newer designs have comparable survivorship and functional outcomes as cemented designs. A long-term (20–30-year) follow-up study of young, active patients who underwent TKA at a mean age of 51 years revealed 70.1 % survivorship without revision. Those who had cementless cruciate-retaining components had two designs, one with 95 % survivability at 12 years and the other with 99 % survivability at 18 years [8]. A Cochrane Review of five randomized, controlled trials with 297 patients revealed that at 2 years postoperatively, cemented TKA fixation demonstrated less displacement than cementless fixation; however, the cemented components went on to have two times the risk of future aseptic loosening compared to cementless fixation [9].

The 2014 Annual Report of the National Joint Registry of England and Wales [10] has also supported that cementless or hybrid fixation with unconstrained fixed and mobile-bearing designs has a similar probability of revision as cemented designs (Fig. 8.4a, b).

The 2014 Annual Report of the Australian Joint Registry reported the same finding with approximately the same cumulative percent revision of 4 % at 10 years. Thus, current data supports the use of cementless fixation, and it may be an advantageous choice in the young, active patient because of the possibility for improved long-term survivorship compared to cemented fixation.

8.5   Bearing Mobility (Fixed versus Mobile)

The primary rationale for using a mobile-bearing TKA design is to reduce wear while affording greater conformity. This sounds like an attractive option for young, active patients; however, the literature has not supported that mobile-bearing knees provide any greater function or better durability than fixed designs. Long et al. found the survivability of five fixed-bearing designs in young, active patients to range from 84 to 100 % at 9–16 years [8]. In 2014, Kim et al. published their 12-year follow-up data on 444 patients who underwent simultaneous bilateral TKA with a single manufacturer's fixed design as well as its mobile-bearing one. They found no significant difference between designs with respect to several activity scores, range of motion, prevalence of aseptic loosening, or survival rate, which was over 97 % for both groups [11]. The 2014 Annual Report of the Australian Registry actually reported a lower cumulative percent revision for fixed-bearing designs throughout their 13 years of reported follow-up. At 10 years, fixed-bearing knees had a 5 % cumulative percent revision compared to 6–7 % among various mobile-bearing designs (Fig. 8.5).

Thus, the current evidence remains convincing that fixed- and mobile-bearing designs afford the same functional outcomes and survivorship.

8.6   Level of Constraint (Cruciate Retaining versus Posterior Stabilized)

The level of constraint in a primary TKA, whether it is cruciate retaining or posterior stabilized (also described as cruciate sacrificing), is another frequent concern of young patients who usually favor preserving as much of their anatomy as possible and may fear mechanically imposed limitations to their motion. A meta-analysis of 130 studies with nearly 10,000 patients with a mean 4-year follow-up of patients who had both types of constraint measured outcomes with a global rating scale [12].

This instrument measured patient outcomes in the domains of pain, function, and range of motion and combined them into a summary scale. Although patients with cruciate-retaining designs had the highest postoperative global scores and greatest global score increase from preoperatively to postoperatively, patients with posterior-stabilized designs had the highest percentage of reported good or excellent outcome (91.7 %), and there was no significant difference in outcomes between the two designs (Fig. 8.6).

The 2013 Annual Report of the American Joint Replacement Registry reported that the majority (59 %) of TKAs done in the United States are posterior stabilized, and there has yet to be proof of inferiority of this design warranting a practice change. In contrast, the 2014 Annual Report of the Australian Registry described a slightly higher rate of cumulative percent revision in their posterior-stabilized TKAs from 1 to 13 years postoperatively (HR 1.21, p <0.001 at 2+ years postoperatively). Nonetheless, there remains insufficient evidence

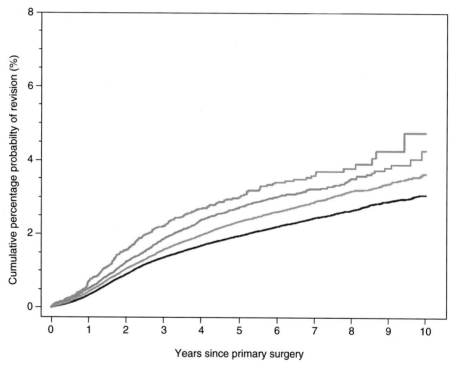

Number at risk

— Unconstrained, fixed	377,653	321,403	264,344	213,010	167,335	125,859	88,296	56,801	34,361	16,083	4,956
— Unconstrained, mobile	27,574	25,517	23,158	20,431	17,099	13,491	9,458	5,681	2,998	1,184	347
— Posterior-stabilised, fixed	141,684	122,228	102,394	83,196	65,192	48,737	33,743	21,372	12,731	6,135	1,872
— Posterior-stabilised, mobile	9,283	8,171	7,102	6,009	4,839	3,749	2,743	1,732	916	340	98

Fig. 8.4 (**a**) Comparison of the Kaplan–Meier cumulative percentage probability estimates of a knee prosthesis first revision for different bearing types at increasing years after the primary surgery with cemented-only fixation (2014 Annual Report of the National Joint Registry of England and Wales). (**b**) Comparison of the Kaplan–Meier cumulative percentage probability estimates of a knee prosthesis first revision for different bearing types at increasing years after the primary surgery with uncemented or hybrid fixation (2014 Annual Report of the National Joint Registry of England and Wales)

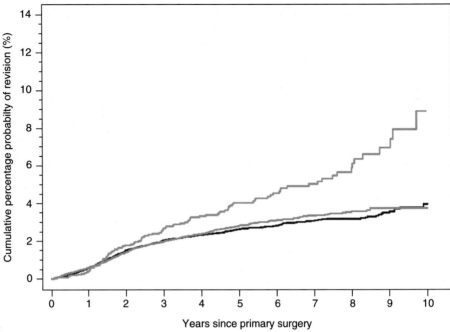

Number at risk											
— Unconstrained, fixed	19,831	18,629	17,113	15,282	12,975	10,107	7,282	4,742	2,997	1,482	462
— Unconstrained, mobile	17,899	16,314	14,269	12,087	9,934	7,845	5,611	3,694	2,274	1,136	348
— Posterior-stabilised, fixed	2,687	2,457	2,205	1,966	1,700	1,353	1,042	724	402	203	66

Fig. 8.4 (continued)

to strongly recommend one level of constraint for young, active patients undergoing TKA.

8.7 Bearing Material

Over the last decade, there has been a trend in knee arthroplasty—largely inspired by the experience with osteolysis in total hip arthroplasty (THA)—that has resulted in decreased utilization of conventional polyethylene inserts in the United States (Fig. 8.7).

Currently, nearly half of tibial inserts are highly cross-linked polyethylene (XLPE), approximately one-third are conventional polyethylene, 10 % are vitamin E infused, and 11 % are unknown. Although the improved wear characteristics of XLPE were proven clearly in THA, it remains a source of debate whether this improved wear profile translates to show favorable

benefit in the very different biomechanical environment of TKA. However, the 2014 Annual Report of the Australian Joint Registry Report shows evidence that XLPE in TKA demonstrates improved performance compared to conventional polyethylene. Cumulative percent revision and osteolysis as a reason for revision are lower in the TKAs with XLPE (Fig. 8.8a, b).

Given these data, it is reasonable to consider XLPE for use in TKA for young, active patients.

8.8 Patellar Resurfacing

Whether to resurface the patella has been a long-standing debate in TKA with wide variability in practice patterns across the world. He et al. performed a meta-analysis of 16 randomized controlled trials from 1966 to 2009 and found that there was no difference in anterior knee pain rate,

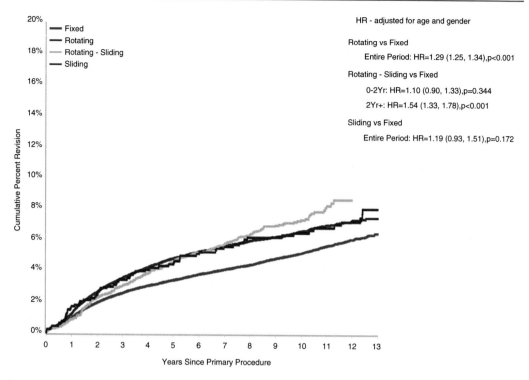

Fig. 8.5 Cumulative percent revision of primary total knee replacement by bearing mobility for patients with primary diagnosis of osteoarthritis (Orthopaedic Association National Joint Replacement Registry. Annual Report. Adelaide: AOA, 2014)

	Mean (Range)*					
	PCL Sparing (n=61)†	ACL and PCL Sacrificing Without PCL Substitution (n=45)†	ACL and PCL Sacrificing With PCL Substitution (n=34)†	ACL and PCL Sacrificing With PCL and Collateral Substitution (n=5)†	Mixed Classes (n=9)†	Total (95%CI)‡ (n=154)†
No. of patients	59.0(13-291)	70.1(11-225)	67.4 (10-182)	28.8 (14-46)	76.4 (14-366)	64.1 (63.1-65.1)
Preoperative global rating score	44.5 (28.0-63.0)	40.2(10.0-64)	46.4 (34.0-0.57.0)	37.9 (21.9-49.0)	45.7 (40-59)	43.5 (41.7-45.3)
Postoperative global rating score	89.3 (79-100)‖	83.6(67.0-92.9)	86.5 (67-94)	79.3 (73.7-87.0)	85.7 (82-94)	86.6 (85.6-87.6)
Difference between preoperative and postoperative global rating score§	46.2 (21.0-68.00)¶	44.4(17-76.0)	40.3(29.0-49.0)	40.7 (26.0-52.0)	41.2 (24-81)	44.0 (41.9-46.1)
Postoperative range of motion	106.8 (65-123)#	98.5 (84-113)	103.1(85-115)	101.3 (96-112)	95.0 (90-115)	102.4 (100.4-104.4)
Patients with good or excellent outcome rating, %	90.4 (68-100)	86.2 (52-100)‖	91.7(79-89)	79.0 (71-94)	92.4 (83-100)	89.3 (88.6-90.0)

Fig. 8.6 Patient outcomes by anatomic classification of prostheses. *ACL* anterior cruciate ligament. *PCL* posterior cruciate ligament (Table 3. *JAMA*, 1994;271(17):1349–57)

knee pain score, American Knee Society score, or function score [13]. The only significant finding was that the reoperation rate was lower in the resurfacing group ($p=0.03$). The arguments against resurfacing are the number of potential negative sequelae: loosening, fragmentation,

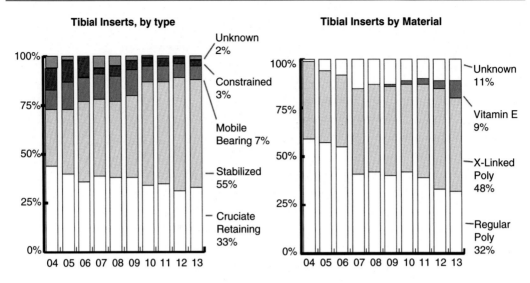

Fig. 8.7 Trend in tibial insert type and material from 2004 to 2013 [14]

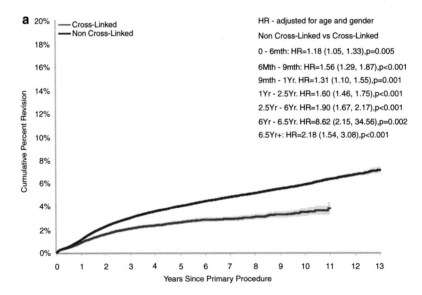

Fig. 8.8 (**a**) Cumulative percent revision of primary total knee replacement by polyethylene bearing surface (Orthopaedic Association National Joint Replacement Registry. Annual Report. Adelaide: AOA, 2014). (**b**)

Cumulative incidence revision diagnosis of primary total knee replacement by polyethylene bearing surface (Orthopaedic Association National Joint Replacement Registry. Annual Report. Adelaide: AOA, 2014)

avascular necrosis, lateral facet pain, stress fracture, acute fracture, late fracture, maltracking, and restricted motion (Fig. 8.9).

The salvage options when these complications are encountered are fraught with poor outcomes, which only become more challenging to manage

when they occur in younger patients who expect higher function and durability from their TKA. Thus, in the young patient, it is reasonable to consider to not resurface the patella. This provides for a faster procedure, lower expense, and lower risk of major complications and reserves

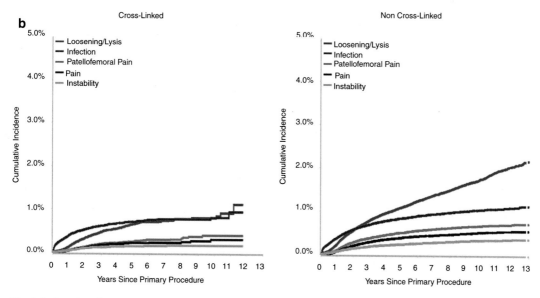

Fig. 8.8 (continued)

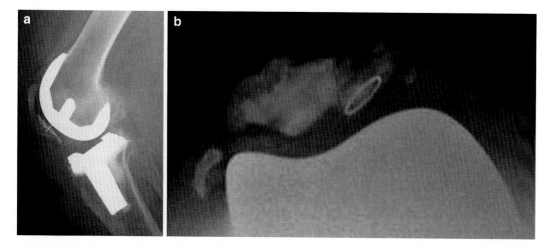

Fig. 8.9 Lateral (**a**) and merchant (**b**) view x-rays demonstrating a fragmented patella and loose patellar component

resurfacing as a relatively easier salvage option in the future.

8.9   Medical Adjuncts

The recent increasing utilization of two medical adjuncts—tranexamic acid and liposomal bupivacaine—in the perioperative care of TKA patients has resulted in improved pain control and decreased blood loss. Especially among young patients, these agents may help facilitate an accelerated postoperative recovery.

Tranexamic acid (TXA) is an antifibrinolytic agent that helps reduce blood loss and ultimately decreases the need for postoperative blood transfusions. A recent study by Whiting et al. has shown that regardless of preoperative hemoglobin level, use of TXA significantly decreases the rate of transfusion by up to eightfold for those with hemoglobin greater than 15 mg/dl and by up to fourfold for those with hemoglobin greater than 11 mg/dl [15]. Consequently, those who did not have to have a transfusion had a significantly shorter length of hospital stay (0.51 compared to 0.69 days). TXA can be administered intravenously or topically, and several randomized controlled trials as well as a meta-analysis have shown that both methods are safe and equally efficacious [16, 17].

Liposomal bupivacaine (Exparel™, Pacira, Inc.) is an extended-release local anesthetic that is administered intraoperatively as a periarticular injection. It has begun to show promise as an effective tool for postoperative pain management. For some surgeons, this has begun to replace the routine use of peripheral nerve blocks, since its use is associated with decreased incidence of falls while providing the same pain relief and perhaps a decreased length of stay [18]. Moreover, a recent study has shown that some patients may experience improved pain scores at rest compared to those with peripheral nerve blocks and significant reduction in opioid use as well as reduction in cost of TKA [19].

8.10   Performance: Quality of Life, Activity Levels, and Return to Work

In looking at the utility of TKA in younger patients from a society perspective, there is substantial economic benefit. A Markov decision analysis published in 2014 revealed that when taking into account earned income, lost wages, and medical costs, the 30-year cost of TKA in a 50-year-old patient afforded nearly a $70,000 cost benefit compared to nonoperative treatment [20]. Although this is a powerful statistic in support of the performance of TKA in young patients, the ability to predict or ensure clinical success and satisfaction for an individual patient is much more challenging. Thus, it is critical to consider the wide variation in reported clinical outcomes and the patient-specific factors that may play a role in predicting the postoperative function and satisfaction for a given patient.

A prospective observational cohort study of 291 patient (331 knees) treated at 25 community practices revealed that of the 92 % for whom there was 2-year follow-up, 88 % of patients were satisfied, 3 % neutral, and 9 % dissatisfied. Those who had maximal improvement in physical composite scores shared several characteristics. They were treated at institutions performing greater than 50 TKAs per year, had better baseline mental health, were older patients, had cruciate-sparing devices, and had worse preoperative function [21].

Nam et al. also reported a 10 % dissatisfaction rate in their single-institution series with a minimum 1 year of follow-up for 661 patients treated with cruciate-retaining TKA. Only 66 % described their knee as feeling "normal," and 54 % complained of residual symptoms or functional deficits. The factors that were most associated with poor outcome were low-income status ($p=0.012$) and female sex (OR 3.13, 95 % CI 1.5–6.4, $P=0.002$) [22].

Undoubtedly, a patient's postoperative satisfaction is linked to their restoration of function, quality of life, and ability to return to work or athletic activities. One of the first age-matched and gender-matched case–control studies to look at the restoration of function post-TKA revealed that there was no difference in function between sexes and both groups had deterioration of function with age. While 52 % of TKA patients had limitations in function compared to 22 % of controls, they had similar function with respect to the following activities: swimming, golfing, and stationary biking. However, the control group had higher functional scores for kneeling, squatting, moving laterally, cutting, carrying loads, stretching, leg strengthening, dancing, gardening, and sexual activity (Fig. 8.10). Only 40 % of functional deficits post-TKA were attributable to aging [23].

Although patients post-TKA experience difficulty with biomechanically demanding tasks compared to controls, some of these limitations may be more of a reflection of patient perception versus reality. Schai et al. showed that this was indeed the case with respect to the task of kneeling. Although 44 % of patients reported they could kneel easily, when supervised, 80 % were observed to kneel easily. And while 14 % reported being unable to kneel, only 4 % were

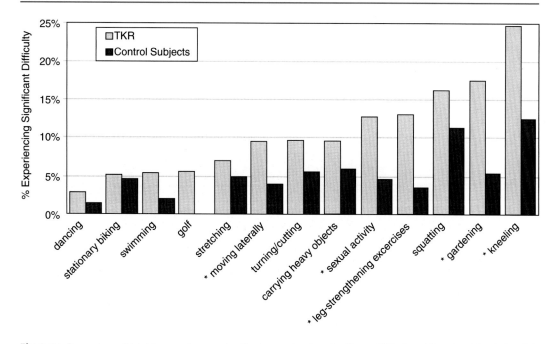

Fig. 8.10 Percentage of total knee replacement patients experiencing significant difficulty with various physical activities compared to age-matched controls (Figure 9. *CORR*, 2005;431:157–65)

noted to have marked difficulty kneeling. Thus, patient perceived ability was significantly lower than their observed ability, and when further questioned, 39 % of patients who reported difficulty cited that it was grounded in fear of harming their prosthesis or some other lack of information about their knee [24].

In counseling a patient preoperatively, it is critical to understand the activities that are important to them and those that they do most frequently. Weiss et al. found that there is a strong correlation between a patient's most prevalent and most important activities [25]. Even when those activities were more demanding (e.g., high flexion, lateral movement, and cutting), a high percentage of patients continued to perform the activity post-TKA even if with limitations (Fig. 8.11).

Improvement in frequency of performance of an activity is often an expectation of patients considering TKA. While the majority of patients are likely to experience an increase in activity level post-TKA, recent data shows that there may be patient-specific parameters that attenuate or negate this effect. Lutzner et al. used an accelerometer to quantify the steps of 97 patients who underwent TKA. Although their number of steps per day increased 1-year post-TKA, they were considerably less when compared with age-matched controls. Further analysis also revealed that body mass index, sex, and comorbidities were independent factors associated with level of activity post-TKA [26]. Consequently, it is especially important for surgeons to help patients establish realistic expectations about their level of activity post-TKA.

Patients who are active preoperatively are even more likely to need counseling about post-TKA athletic activity. These patients are usually most interested in understanding not only the impact of TKA on their ability to return to sport but also the sport impact on their TKA. A systematic review of athletic activity after lower limb arthroplasty has shown that 54–98 % return to sport. And those who return tend to have increased preoperative activity levels, lower age, male sex, lower BMI, and no other joint pain [27]. Patients who underwent unicompartmental knee arthroplasty were more active than those who underwent TKA. There was also no correlation with activity level and early revision rates;

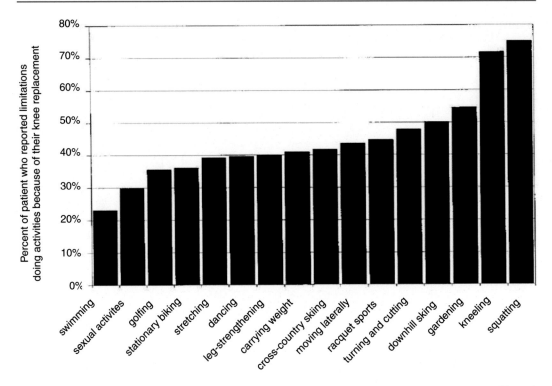

Fig. 8.11 Percentage of patients who reported limitations doing activities because of their knee replacement (Figure 3. *CORR*, 2002;404:172–88)

however, a few studies showed increased wear with increased activity levels.

For the majority of young patients considering TKA, the ability to return to work is an essential component in the final decision-making process or the timing of TKA. A recent systematic review of both hip and knee arthroplasty patients analyzed the outcome for 649 patients who underwent TKA. Return to work by 3–6 months was achieved by 71–83 % of patients by 3–6 months, and the average time to return to work ranged from 8 to 12 weeks. The factors that related to work status after TKA included sociodemographic, health, and job characteristics [28].

8.11   Case Examples

Case 1: Aseptic Femoral Loosening

An active 56-year-old man was treated with primary total knee arthroplasty in 2009 for osteoarthritis with a varus deformity and flexion contracture. The implant used was a Zimmer NexGen Legacy posterior-stabilized (LPS) system (Warsaw, Indiana). He did very well for 3 years until he began to develop a progressive varus deformity and instability with medial knee pain and recurrent effusions. At his pre-revision examination, he was noted to have a +2 effusion, range of motion from full extension to 100° of flexion, 3+ LCL with a soft end point, and a 1+ MCL with a hard end point. X-rays revealed pseudo-varus alignment and medial polyethylene wear (Fig. 8.12).

Intraoperatively, extensive posteromedial wear of the insert was noted and the femoral component was noted to be loose. Patient was revised to a constrained condylar prosthesis. He was able to return to his active lifestyle.

Case 2: Tibial Post Fracture

An active 58-year-old man with a body mass index (BMI) of 33 was treated with primary total

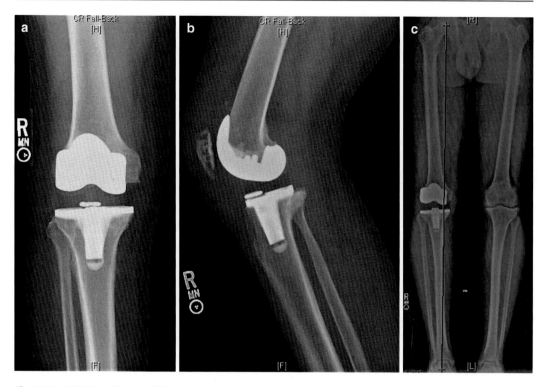

Fig. 8.12 AP (**a**) and lateral (**b**) knee x-rays demonstrating medial polyethylene wear without obvious evidence of component loosening. Full-length standing x-ray (**c**) demonstrates varus alignment

knee arthroplasty in 2002 for posttraumatic arthrosis. The implant used was cemented and posterior stabilized. He did well until 8 years postoperatively when after performing leg extensions with 90 lb of weight, he developed pain, swelling, and instability. Upon evaluation in the clinic, his knee had a large effusion with range of motion from a few degrees of hyperextension to 110° of flexion. There was no obvious varus, valgus, or flexion instability. His posterior drawer was +3 with a soft end point. Postoperative x-rays indicated satisfactory component alignment (Fig. 8.13).

Intraoperatively, the tibial post was found to have fractured with evidence of post wear but no obvious oxidative damage (Fig. 8.14).

Retrieval analysis with scanning electron microscopy demonstrated that fatigue cracks had propagated at the post base from both the anterior and posterior directions and likely led to ultimate fracture from a single overload event [29]. The patient was treated with tibial insert exchange. He maintains an active lifestyle.

Take-Home Points

- TKA should be considered for younger, active patients with osteoarthritis.
- TKA should only be offered after nonoperative treatments fail.
- Cementless fixation should be considered.
- XLPE and oxidatively stabilized PE should be considered.
- No differences with mobile-bearing or constrained components.
- No resurfacing patella should be considered.
- Critical to set expectations for pain relief, improvement in function, and durability.

Fig. 8.13 AP (**a**) and lateral (**b**) knee x-rays demonstrating acceptable component positioning

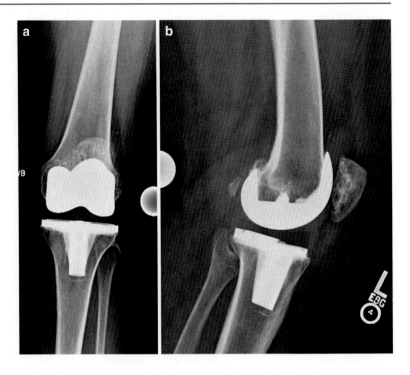

References

1. Australian Orthopaedic Association National Joint Replacement Registry. Annual Report. 2014. www.aoa.org.au.
2. Sharkey PF, Hozack WJ, Rothman RH, et al. Why are total knee arthroplasties failing today? Clin Orthop Relat Res. 2002;404:7–13.
3. Bozic KJ, Kurtz SM, Lau E, et al. The epidemiology of revision total knee arthroplasty in the United States. Clin Orthop Relat Res. 2010;468:45–58.
4. Sharkey PF, Lichstein PM, Chao S, et al. Why are total knee arthroplasties failing today—has anything changed after 10 years? J Arthroplasty. 2014;29:1774–8.
5. Schroer WC, Berend KR, Lombardi AV, et al. Why are total knees failing today? Etiology of total knee revision in 2010 and 2011. J Arthroplasty. 2013;28(1):116–9.
6. Le DH, Goodman SB, Maloney WJ, et al. Current modes of failure in TKA: infection, instability and stiffness predominate. Clin Orthop Relat Res. 2014; 472:2197–200.
7. Bozic KJ, Lau E, Ong K, et al. Risk factors for early revision after primary TKA in medicare patients. Clin Orthop Relat Res. 2014;472:232–7.
8. Long WJ, Bryce CD, Hollenbeak CS, et al. Total knee replacement in young, active patients: long-term follow-up and functional outcome. J Bone Joint Surg Am. 2014;96(18):e159.

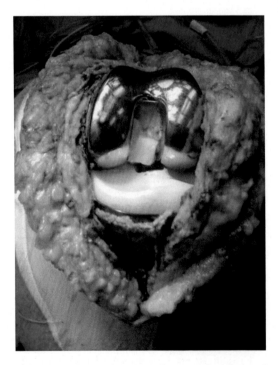

Fig. 8.14 Intraoperative photo demonstrating fractured tibial post

9. Nakama GY, Almeida GJM, Lira N, et al. Cemented, cementless or hybrid fixation options in total knee arthroplasty for osteoarthritis and other non-traumatic diseases. Cochrane Database Syst Rev. 2012;(10):CD006193. doi:10.1002/14651858.CD006193.pub2.

10. National Joint Registry for England, Wales and Northern Ireland. 11th Annual Report. 2014. www.njrreports.org.uk.

11. Kim YH, Park JW, Kim JS. Long-term clinical outcomes and survivorship of press-fit condylar sigma fixed-bearing and mobile-bearing total knee prostheses in the same patient. J Bone Joint Surg Am. 2014; 96(19):e168.

12. Callahan CM, Drake BG, Heck DA, et al. Patient outcomes following tricompartmental total knee replacement: a meta-analysis. JAMA. 1994;271:1349–57.

13. He JY, Jiang LS, Dai LY. Is patellar resurfacing superior than nonresurfacing in TKA? A meta-analysis of randomized trials. Knee. 2011;18(3):137–44.

14. Orthopaedic Network News. 2014;25(3):13.

15. Whiting DR, Duncan CM, Sierra RJ, et al. Tranexamic acid benefits total joint arthroplasty patients regardless of preoperative hemoglobin value. J Arthroplasty. 2015. http://dx.doi.org/10.1016/j.arth.2015.05.050.

16. Shemshaki H, Nourian SM, Nourain N, et al. One step closer to sparing total blood loss and transfusion rate in total knee arthroplasty: a meta-analysis or different methods of tranexamic acid administration. Arch Orthop Trauma Surg. 2015;135(4):573–88.

17. Gomez-Barrena E, Ortega-Andreu M, Padilla-Eguiluz NG, et al. Topical intra-articular compared with intravenous tranexamic acid to reduce blood loss in primary total knee replacement: a double-blind, randomized, controlled, noninferiority clinical trial. Bone Joint Surg Am. 2014;96(23):1937–44.

18. Surdam JW, Baynes NT, Arce BR. The use of exparel (liposomal bupivacaine) to manage postoperative pain in unilateral total knee arthroplasty patients. J Arthroplasty. 2015;30(2):325–9.

19. Springer BD. Transition from nerve blocks to periarticular injections and emerging techniques in total joint arthroplasty. Am J Orthop. 2014;43 Suppl 10:6–9.

20. Bedair H, Cha TD, Hansen VJ. Economic benefit to society at large of total knee arthroplasty in younger patients. A Markov analysis. J Bone Joint Surg Am. 2014;96(2):119–26.

21. Heck DA, Robinson RL, Partridge CM, et al. Patient outcomes after knee replacement. Clin Orthop Relat Res. 1998;356:93–110.

22. Nam D, Nunley RM, Barrack RL. Patient dissatisfaction following total knee replacement. A growing concern? Bone Joint J. 2014;96-B(Suppl A):96–100.

23. Noble PC, Gordon MJ, Weiss JM, et al. Does total knee replacement restore normal knee function? Clin Orthop Relat Res. 2005;431:157–65.

24. Schai PA, Gibbon AJ, Scott RD. Kneeling ability after total knee arthroplasty: perception and reality. Clin Orthop Relat Res. 1999;367:195–200.

25. Weiss JM, Noble PC, Conditt MA, et al. What functional activities are important to patients with knee replacements? Clin Orthop Relat Res. 2002;404:172–88.

26. Lutzner C, Kirschner S, Lutzner J. Patient activity after TKA depends on patient-specific parameters. Clin Orthop Relat Res. 2014;472:3933–40.

27. Jassim SS, Douglas SL, Haddad FS. Athletic activity after lower limb arthroplasty. Bone Joint J. 2014; 96-B:923–7.

28. Tilbury C, Schaasberg W, Pleview JW, et al. Return to work after total hip and knee arthroplasty: a systematic review. Rheumatology. 2014;53:512–25.

29. Ansari F, Chang J, Huddleston JI, et al. Fractography and oxidative analysis of gamma inert sterilized posterior-stabilized tibial insert post fractures: a report of two cases. Knee. 2013;20(6):609–13.

New and Evolving Surgical Techniques

9

Willem van der Merwe

Contents

9.1 Introduction

As a result of increasing life expectancies, continuing physical careers, lifestyles into later life, and rising obesity levels, the number of younger patients presenting with osteoarthritis (OA) of the knee is increasing. When conservative management options have been exhausted, the challenge for the orthopaedic surgeon is to offer a procedure that will relieve symptoms and allow a return to a high level of function but not compromise future surgery.

Young patients are looking for alternatives that can give them back their activity without requiring surgical procedures that are irreversible or may have complications that can really take them down a path of multiple surgeries and poor outcomes.

The number of young patients seeking medical consultation for symptoms relating to osteoarthritis (OA) of the knee is increasing [1]. This is thought to be due to a combination of factors [2]. Longer life expectancy also means that the proportion of the population continuing physically demanding careers and sporting lifestyles into their fifth, sixth, and even seventh decades is increasing [3]. In addition to these risks, there are rising levels of obesity and there is clear evidence that the risk of OA is increased with obesity. Coinciding with the increasing rates of OA are patient expectations that a return to previous levels of activity should be possible following injury or trauma.

This chapter discusses two techniques that are certainly not new concepts but are new and evolving

W. van der Merwe
Department of Orthopaedic Surgery SSISA,
Sport Science Institute of SA,
Boundary Rd, Newlands,
Cape Town 7700, South Africa
e-mail: willem@ssoc.co.za

© ISAKOS 2016
D.A. Parker (ed.), *Management of Knee Osteoarthritis in the Younger, Active Patient:
An Evidence-Based Practical Guide for Clinicians*, DOI 10.1007/978-3-662-48530-9_9

developments of older ideas. These techniques do not change the morphology of the bones as there are no bone cuts and are known as interpositional and distraction or unloading arthroplasty. The concept of preserving the native knee whilst relieving pain and improving function is potentially appealing to this population of young athletes, and by using new technology and better materials, these concepts have once again become an area of interest for clinicians.

9.2 Interpositional Arthroplasty

Interpositional implants were developed in order to manage pain and increase function in a way that preserves bone and delays the need for a knee replacement. Both biologic and metal interpositional implant/arthroplasty procedures are currently available for the treatment of unicompartmental OA. In biologic interpositional arthroplasty, an allograft meniscus is employed in the transplantation, as was covered in Chap. 3.

Metal interpositional arthroplasty procedures were first developed in the 1950s by MacIntosh and McKeever. This procedure was practically abandoned when joint replacement arthroplasty with methyl methacrylate was introduced. However, the concept of a metal interpositional arthroplasty has recently seen a resurgence with the development of a prosthetic device marketed as UniSpacer. The US FDA approved UniSpacer in 2000 with the purpose of restoring alignment of the knee and thereby improving pain and function. A second interpositional device, the iForma, also came to the market recently through a 510(k) exemption. As opposed to the mass-produced "off-the-shelf" UniSpacer, which is only available in 24 sizes, iForma is custom manufactured, using MRI scans, to be fitted specifically for an individual patient. These new devices are thought to restore alignment and stability by replacing missing articular and meniscal cartilage with a metallic implant.

UniSpacer can be thought of as a mobile McKeever or MacIntosh implant. Instead of an attempt at fixation to the tibial plateau via a keel or roughened undersurface, UniSpacer is designed to translate freely on the tibial plateau

as determined by the conforming articulation of its top surface with the femoral condyle. The insertion of the implant does not require any bone resection or any mechanical fixation to the tibial plateau for proper function. The iForma implant is a self-fixating version of a metallic hemiarthroplasty as previously described by MacIntosh and McKeever. By using three-dimensional sizing software, an individual medial or lateral interpositional implant is generated based on the MRI data of the affected knee joint. The generated device is then implanted using a minimally invasive technique with a 5 cm incision. iForma is characterized by a highly constraining undersurface that exactly mirrors the tibial plateau with resultant self-fixation on the tibia. The implant's individual adaptation to each patient's respective surface geometry is thought to provide a functionally stable fit.

Whilst the proponents of these devices had suggested they would provide a simple, joint-preserving technique to relieve arthritic pain, the actual results have been somewhat disappointing. The UK National Institute for Health and Clinical Excellence (NICE) published a rapid systematic review (level of evidence 1) investigating the efficacy/effectiveness of magnetic resonance imaging-designed unicompartmental interpositional implants (*at present, the only device investigated has been iForma*) to treat OA of the knee. This systematic review identified one published study [4] and incorporated two sets of unpublished data submitted by two orthopaedic consultants in the UK. The additional unpublished data from 84 and 60 patients only reported on the occurrence of revision, which was 5 % and 7 %, respectively. Based on this rapid systematic review, NICE issued clinical guidelines [1] in September 2009 stating that current evidence on the safety and efficacy of individual magnetic resonance imaging-designed unicompartmental interpositional implant insertion for knee OA was inadequate in quality and quantity, and as such, the procedure should be considered experimental.

In December 2008, the American Academy of Orthopaedic Surgeons (AAOS) also published a clinical practice guideline on the treatment of OA of the knee (nonarthroplasty). With regard to interpositional implants, the organization suggested, based on the outcome of a study conducted by Sisto et al. [5] and the Australian Joint Replacement Registry, that free-floating interpositional devices, that is, the UniSpacer, should not be used for patients with symptomatic unicompartmental OA of the knee. Therefore, this device cannot be recommended for routine use in knee osteoarthritis.

The third implant in the interpositional arthroplasty category is the "NUsurface" implant which is an artificial polycarbonate-urethane meniscus device. Computational-experimental approach for the design of a free-floating polycarbonate-urethane (PCU) meniscal implant was used in the original design [6]. Validated 3D finite element (FE) models of the knee and PCU-based implant were analysed under physiological loads. Several models of the implant, some including embedded reinforcement fibres, were tested. An optimal implant configuration was then selected based on the ability to restore pressure distribution in the knee, manufacturability, and long-term safety. Investigation using a sheep model showed that the nondegradable anatomically shaped artificial meniscal implant, composed of Kevlar-reinforced polycarbonate-urethane (PCU), could prevent progressive cartilage degeneration following complete meniscectomy [7]. Another pilot study examined the kinematics of a knee implanted with the artificial polycarbonate-urethane meniscus device. The static kinematic behaviour of the implant was compared to the natural medial meniscus of the non-operated knee. A second goal was to evaluate the motion pattern, the radial displacement, and the deformation of the meniscal implant. The implant, indicated for medial meniscus replacement, had no influence on femoral rollback and tibiofemoral contact points, thus suggesting that the joint maintains its static kinematic properties after implantation. Radial displacement and meniscal height were not different, but anteroposterior movement was slightly different between the implant and the normal meniscus [8]. The NUsurface meniscal implant is currently in medical trials to investigate its effectiveness and safety.

These free-floating devices have many potential advantages but so far, no clinical study has confirmed clinical effectiveness and low -complications. The NUsurface can potentially address some of the problems experienced with the metal implants because the polycarbonate is more forgiving and can shape to the femoral condyle more readily. Most commonly, there is articular cartilage wear, so when the interpositional device is inserted, this loss of cartilage is accounted for and the alignment of the knee is theoretically being restored in extension. However, when the knee is flexed, there is less wear posteriorly and therefore a smaller gap, but the thickness of the implant is constant and over-stuffing can lead to pain in flexion or dislocation. Hopefully, the forgiveness of the polycarbonate can overcome this issue. The results of the current medical trial will need to be reviewed before we will know whether this technology will provide a solution for patients.

9.3 Distraction Arthroplasty

Few options are available for treatment of end-stage knee OA and none have clearly been shown to affect the natural history of the condition. Removal of pain by replacing the destroyed joint with an endoprosthesis is the currently accepted treatment option for severe knee OA. Consequently, the number of total knee prostheses is exponentially increasing in the Western world and causes major economic burden. Over 40 % of all knee replacements and up to 44 % of all total knee revision procedures are performed in patients aged under 65. Importantly, the procedure has a higher risk of failure in younger patients. As such, development of alternative treatment strategies for severe knee OA, specifically those that can postpone a first prosthesis, is constantly being sought.

Joint distraction is a surgical procedure in which the two opposing joint surfaces are gradually separated to a certain extent for a certain period of time. Initially, joint distraction was used in the treatment of joint malalignment and joint contracture. An external fixation frame was used to actively reposition the joint and to increase the range of motion. Distraction was performed to prevent damage (compression) of the joint cartilage during the forced repositioning. In some of these patients, OA was present in the treated joint and an unexpected clinical improvement of the OA was observed. These clinical observations led to a proof-of-concept study examining the benefit of joint distraction, by treating young patients with severe ankle OA. Two-thirds of patients treated for 3 months with joint distraction experienced significant clinical benefits for a period of up to 10 years. Based on preliminary radiographic outcome in a limited number of patients, it was suggested that joint distraction may lead to tissue structure modification as well. Distraction therapy might be perceived as a burdensome treatment for patients because they experience 2 months of joint stiffness and potential pin tract pain/infection during the distraction period. Despite these side effects, the clinical benefit appeared worth the "investment", as reported by all patients. Moreover, alternative surgical interventions such as osteotomy may also involve a lengthy recovery and associated inconvenience.

One of the most impressive and maybe unexpected results was that the denuded bone areas (dABp) were diminished and filled with tissue that has the same signal intensity as cartilage, when estimated by MR imaging. This challenges the dogma that intrinsic cartilage repair is not possible, although it is difficult to postulate that this effect is solely due to an increased matrix synthesis of resident chondrocytes. As such, it is postulated that resident mesenchymal stem cells (MSCs) in the joint are important for intra-articular repair activity. Contribution appears to consist of metabolic stimulation of existing chondrocytes or differentiation in an osteogenic manner into new chondrocytes. Hydrostatic dynamic pressure (1–10 kPa), as measured intra-articular during knee and ankle joint distraction when applied in vitro, can stimulate MSCs in coculture with cartilage, leading to cartilage matrix synthesis.

Developing this concept, Ochi et al. described an articulated distraction arthroplasty device for the treatment of OA of the knee [9]. The uniqueness of their device was that it was articulated, allowing knee flexion. Kajiwara et al. [10] reported on the success of a similar device in treating cartilage damage in an animal model. In this case, distraction arthroplasty was performed with the patient under lumbar anaesthesia. Arthroscopy was used to examine the cartilage surfaces, menisci, and ligaments in all cases. Bone marrow stimulation was then performed under arthroscopy. After the external devices were removed, follow-up arthroscopy revealed that in all cases, the regions treated with the bone marrow stimulation procedure were covered with newly formed tissues. Although one case had a superficial skin infection around the insertion of the pin at the tibia, no patient had any major complications such as nerve palsy or deep infection. Clinical improvements were also seen, with improved outcome scores, pain, range of motion, and joint space. Ochi has now developed a distraction device that uses a magnetic force to distract the joint more evenly through full ROM. This device can be used to distract the lateral compartment but at this stage is just at the cadaveric analysis stage, and therefore, this concept is still in development [11].

Distraction arthroplasty has therefore shown promise in promoting regeneration of the joint surface, most likely fibrocartilage, in patients with OA. One significant problem with this technique is the invasiveness of the distraction device. However, the pins are extra-articular and when removed, there is no residual metal in the knee that may compromise future surgery. This concept is still very much in the development phase, but the initial promising findings suggest that this field will continue to develop in the future. In combination with better biological methods, this may provide clinicians with techniques to help restore cartilage in the setting of generalized osteoarthritis and positively affect the natural history of the condition.

Along these lines, a new device marketed as the "KineSpring® Knee Implant System" (Moximed, Inc, Hayward, CA, USA) is an implantable, extra-articular, extra-capsular prosthesis intended to alleviate knee OA-related symptoms by reducing medial knee compartment loading whilst overcoming the limitations of traditional joint-unloading therapies. Preclinical and clinical studies have demonstrated excellent prosthesis durability, substantial reductions in medial compartment

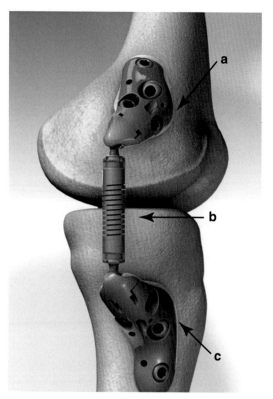

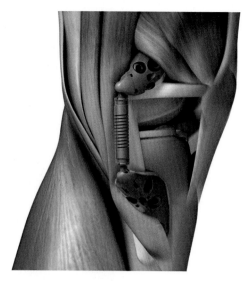

Fig. 9.2 Schematic drawing of the KineSpring® Knee Implant System (Moximed, Inc, Hayward, CA, USA) in relation to key anatomical structures

Fig. 9.1 Compohe KineSpring® Knee Implant System (Moximed, Inc, Hayward, CA, USA). (a) Femoral base, (b) load absorber spring, (c) tibial base

and total joint loads, and clinically important improvements in OA-related pain and function. This system consists of titanium alloy low-contact femoral and tibial bases and a cobalt chrome alloy absorber that reduces the load carried by the diseased medial compartment of the knee joint during the stance phase of gait (Fig. 9.1). The low-contact femoral and tibial bases are affixed to the bone with compression and locking screws. The bases are designed with three undersurface stand-offs that allow the bases to contact the bone at discrete locations without requiring elevation or removal of the periosteum. The load absorber resides in the subcutaneous tissue on the medial aspect of the knee and is positioned superficial to the medial collateral ligament [12]. This single-spring absorber is designed to compress and absorb up to 29 lb of joint load during knee extension and to lengthen and become passive during knee flexion (Fig. 9.2).

Concerns with this device include the durability and effectiveness of the spring mechanism and the potential for soft tissue irritation. The device is still in the clinical trial phase, but the initial clinical experience seems promising. Composite data from three clinical trials [13–15] in 99 patients with 17 months mean follow-up suggest excellent safety and effectiveness. All devices were successfully implanted and activated with no intraoperative complications. Statistically significant mean improvements of 56, 50, and 38 % were observed for Western Ontario and McMaster Universities Osteoarthritis Index (WOMAC) Pain, Function, and Stiffness scores, respectively (all $P < 0.001$). WOMAC clinical success rates were 77.8 % for pain, 77.8 % for function, and 68.7 % for stiffness. The worldwide experience with the current generation KineSpring System has yielded favourable safety and durability outcomes with only 12 (8 %) patients undergoing device removal during follow-up for soft tissue impingement [6], return of OA symptoms [4], or deep infection [2]. Only one patient in this cohort was converted to arthroplasty after removal of the KineSpring device. Typical pretreatment and follow-up radiographs from this worldwide experience are shown in Fig. 9.3.

This type of device certainly appears to show promise and merits further investigation. Two

Fig. 9.3 (a) Preoperative anteroposterior radiograph showing pronounced osteoarthritis of the medial compartment. (b) The KineSpring® Knee Implant System (Moximed, Inc, Hayward, CA, USA) at 2 years post-implant

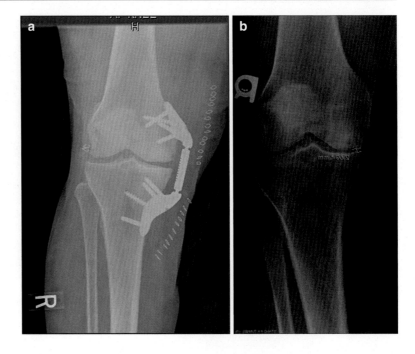

clinical trials are currently underway to further evaluate the safety and effectiveness of the KineSpring System. The GOAL study (NCT01610505) 25 is a prospective, nonrandomized, controlled postmarket study comparing outcomes of 225 patients treated with the KineSpring System or high tibial valgus osteotomy. The first patient was enrolled in June 2012 and enrolment is expected to continue through 2013. A single-arm FDA-approved Investigational Device Exemption study ([SOAR] NCT01738165) [16] with 30 patients began enrolment in December 2012. Patient enrolment is anticipated to continue through mid-2013; the primary outcome will be evaluated at 2 years, and patients will be followed for 5 years post-treatment. The results of these clinical trials should help in deciding on the effectiveness and safety of these devices and in defining the appropriate indications.

9.4   Summary

Management of OA in the young active patient presents a significant challenge for the clinician who is trying to find appropriate options for patients who want to be active and not compromise their lifestyle, but avoid more invasive procedures such as arthroplasty. Procedures that

are less invasive such as interposition arthroplasty and distraction or unloading arthroplasty potentially provide these less invasive options for patients that may not only improve symptoms but also positively affect the natural history of their condition.

Many of these devices, despite apparently well-considered designs, have ultimately had high failure rates when applied clinically. For this reason, any new technology needs to undergo appropriate scientific testing and clinical trials before introduction to the general community. The results of current clinical trials underway for devices discussed in this chapter will be awaited with interest. If early promising results translate to good results in clinical trials, then these devices may provide a useful addition to treatment options for these patients. Given the scope of this problem, it is inevitable that new technologies will continue to emerge with every year.

References

1. National Institute for Health and Clinical Excellence. *National* Collaborating Centre for Chronic Conditions Osteoarthritis: national clinical guideline for care and management in adults. London: NICE; 2008.

2. Woolf AD, Pfleger B. Burden of major musculoskeletal conditions. Bull WHO 2003;81:646–56. Feeley
BT, Gallo RA, Shermsan S, Williams RJ. Management
of osteoarthritis of the knee in the active patient. J Am
Acad Orthop Surg. 2010;18:406–16.
3. McLellan F. Obesity rising to alarming levels around
the world. Lancet. 2002;359:1412.
4. Koeck FX, Luring C, Handel M, Tingart M, Grifka J,
Beckmann J. Prospective single-arm, multi-center
trial of a patient-specific interpositional knee implant:
early clinical results. Open Orthop J. 2011;5:37–43.
5. Sisto DJ, Mitchell IL. Unispacer arthroplasty of the
knee. J Bone Joint Surg Am. 2005;87(8):1706–11.
6. Elsner JJ, Portnoy S, Zur G, Guilak F, Shterling A,
Linder-Ganz E. Design of a free-floating polycarbonate-
urethane meniscal implant using finite element model-
ing and experimental validation. J Biomech Eng.
2010;132(9):095001.
7. Zur G, Linder-Ganz E, Elsner JJ, Shani J, Brenner O,
Agar G, Hershman EB, Arnoczky SP, Guilak F,
Shterling A. Chondroprotective effects of a polycarbonate-
urethane meniscal implant: histopathological results in
a sheep model. Knee Surg Sports Traumatol Arthrosc.
2011;19(2):255–63.
8. De Coninck T, Elsner JJ, Linder-Ganz E, Cromheecke
M, Shemesh M, Huysse W, Verdonk R, Verstraete K,
Verdonk P. In-vivo evaluation of the kinematic behav-
ior of an artificial medial meniscus implant: a pilot
study using open-MRI. Clin Biomech (Bristol, Avon).
2014;29(8):898–905.
9. Deie M, Ochi M, Adachi N, Kajiwara R, Kanaya A. A
new articulated distraction arthroplasty device for
treatment of the osteoarthritic knee joint: a preliminary report. Arthroscopy. 2007;23(8):L833–8.
10. Kajiwara R, Ishida O, Kawasaki K, Adachi N,
Yasunaga Y, Ochi M. Effective repair of a fresh
osteochondral defect in the rabbit knee joint by articulated joint distraction following subchondral drilling.
J Orthop Res. 2005;23:909–15.
11. Kamei G, Ochi M, Okuhara A, Fujimiya M, Deie M,
Adachi N, Nakamae A, Nakasa T, Ohkawa S,
Takazawa K, Eguchi A, Katou T, Takada T, Usman
MA. A new distraction arthroplasty device using
magnetic force; a cadaveric study. Clin Biomech
(Bristol, Avon). 2013;28(4):423–8. doi:10.1016/j.
clinbiomech.2013.02.003.
12. Gabriel SM, Clifford AG, Maloney WJ, O'Connell
MK, Tornetta III P. Unloading the OA knee with a
novel implant system. J Appl Biomech. 2012;29(6):
647–54.
13. Moximed, Inc. Safety and feasibility of a load bypass
knee support system (LBKSS) for the treatment of
osteoarthritis. Camperdown: The Australian New
Zealand Clinical Trials Registry; 2008. anzctr.org.au
[website on the Internet]. Accessed 7 Mar 2013.
14. Moximed, Inc. A multi-center, open-label, interven-
tional study of patients with medial compartment knee
osteoarthritis (OA) treated with the KineSpring®System.
Camperdown: The Australian New Zealand Clinical
Trials Registry; 2009. anzctr.org.au [website on the
Internet]. Accessed 7 Mar 2013.
15. Moximed, Inc. The treatment of medial compartmental knee osteoarthritis (OA) symptoms with the
KineSpring™ Unicompartmental Knee Arthroplasty
(UKA) System. London: Current Controlled Trials
Ltd; 2009. controlled-trials.com [website on the
Internet]. Accessed 7 Mar 2013.
16. Moximed, Inc. Pilot study of the KineSpring® System
to evaluate symptom relief in patients with medial
knee osteoarthritis (SOAR). Bethesda: US National
Library of Medicine; 2012. ClinicalTrials.gov [web-
site on the Internet]. Accessed 7 Mar 2013.

Conclusions

10

David A. Parker

Osteoarthritis of the knee joint encompasses a spectrum of pathology ranging from early chondral damage and degenerative meniscal pathology to more advanced well-established "bone-on-bone" disease. Deciding on the management of elderly patients with osteoarthritis is a relatively straightforward process, given that joint replacement will usually successfully address advanced disease and meet these patients' expectations. However, younger patients with osteoarthritis have different activity profiles and expectations, and increasingly commonly, physicians are faced with relatively young patients who are affected by painful joints resulting from articular cartilage pathology, ranging from early wear to well-established osteoarthritis. These patients are typically active and wishing to remain active in sports, work, and family life, and are less accepting of the restrictions placed on them by osteoarthritis. In the absence of a cure for osteoarthritis, it is vitally important that the treating physician has a comprehensive knowledge of the options for managing

these patients and allowing them to continue an active lifestyle.

There are many options for management of osteoarthritis in these patients, and in modern society, there are many treatments promoted, through either popular media or direct promotion to patients and clinicians. Given the common nature of the problem, there are obviously strong market forces driving this promotion since any treatment that becomes popular will generate huge ongoing income for the provider. It can be difficult for patients, and even sometimes for clinicians, to sort through the literature and other promotional material to decide which treatments actually have scientific merit from an appropriate evidence base. Clearly, physicians can only provide patients with optimal management if they have an up-to-date knowledge of the available treatment options, the evidence base available for each, and the appropriate timing and indications for each treatment. The purpose of this book has been to create a resource that provides physicians with a practical guide to managing these patients in a comprehensive evidence-based manner.

The chapters of this book have covered the pathogenesis and natural history of osteoarthritis, as well as the nonoperative and operative approaches to the condition. Osteoarthritis is a condition that has been widely studied in recent times, with an improved understanding of its aetiology and progression. As discussed in the first chapter, despite this greater understanding,

D.A. Parker, MBBS(Hons), BMedSci, FRACS
North Shore Knee Clinic, Sydney, NSW, Australia

Sydney Orthopaedic Research Institute, Chatswood, NSW, Australia

University of Sydney, Sydney, NSW, Australia

Queensland University of Technology, Brisbane, QLD, Australia
e-mail: dparker@sydneyortho.com.au

© ISAKOS 2016
D.A. Parker (ed.), *Management of Knee Osteoarthritis in the Younger, Active Patient: An Evidence-Based Practical Guide for Clinicians*, DOI 10.1007/978-3-662-48530-9_10

there are still many areas that are yet to be clearly defined, which will therefore be the subject of ongoing study. Osteoarthritis is clearly not simply loss of articular cartilage, but a disease that affects the joint globally, with wide variation in the clinical response between patients. There are definite factors associated with its development, including a history of injury, family history, and obesity, but the specific "recipe" that defines and predicts the risk profile for the development and progression of osteoarthritis for each individual is still something being defined. At this stage, it should, however, be possible for clinicians to counsel patients regarding the aetiology of their osteoarthritis, the severity of their disease, the risk and rate of likely progression, and the modifiable risk factors that they may be able to address. This fundamental understanding of the condition by the clinician, and imparted to the patient, is critical in the successful management of each patient.

Nonsurgical management of osteoarthritis should in most cases be the first option discussed with patients, with surgery usually reserved for those patients for whom nonsurgical management has not been able to satisfactorily manage their condition. Even in patients for whom surgery has been elected, appropriate ongoing nonsurgical management usually remains an important supplement to their treatment. It is often difficult for the physician to advise patients on nonsurgical management, as patients will often feel that they need to have "something done" to address their problem and will perceive a recommendation for nonsurgical management as an indication that nothing actually can be done. This is probably a reflection of the common approach to nonoperative management, often involving suggestions of various options for patients to self-manage, which can lead to confusion for the patient and a subsequent inefficient application of the treatments. The chapter on nonsurgical management of OA has comprehensively reviewed the many options available for treatment, which is a list that will continue to rapidly evolve as more options arise with considerable regularity. Understanding the evidence base and indications for these options is important, but

equally important is the effective application of these options for each patient.

The concept of a coordinated multidisciplinary approach to nonsurgical management is one that has met with success in many centres and should certainly improve the effectiveness of nonsurgical treatment. In such a programme, a central coordinator assesses each patient's condition, decides which treatment modalities are likely to be most effective, and then coordinates the various treatments for the patients. This ensures the necessary understanding and compliance for each patient, and subsequent follow-up and review with the initial coordinator allow positive feedback for the patient and modification of the programme as necessary. With time, the patient's understanding increases, and they become more adept at self-management. In this way, the nonsurgical management of OA becomes a more proactive and defined process, which each patient can clearly understand and appreciate the benefits of. In the future, these multidisciplinary clinics should become the norm for nonsurgical management and, with increasing experience, should be able to become better defined, better managed, and ultimately more effective.

Surgical management in OA is usually reserved for patients for whom nonsurgical management has become ineffective or is judged unlikely to be of any significant benefit. There are a spectrum of surgical options that have been used in the management of OA, and with time and experience, it has become possible to more clearly define the effectiveness of each treatment and better refine the indications for each patient. This increased understanding has led to changes in practice in recent times, for example, in the use of arthroscopic debridement in the management of OA. With the advent of arthroscopic surgery, debridement of arthritic knees and associated pathology such as degenerative meniscal tears became routine practice. However, over the last decade, several studies, as well as general clinical experience, have demonstrated that this procedure has little, if any, benefit and, as a result, should rarely be performed. There are certain instances for which arthroscopic surgery in the presence of arthritis may be appropriate, and these have been outlined clearly in the fourth chapter of this text.

One area for which surgery is appropriate is in preservation of the meniscus. The third chapter of this text has clearly outlined the function of the meniscus and its importance in prevention of osteoarthritis. Therefore, whilst debridement of meniscal tears has been the more common procedure, and should likely decrease in frequency with a more evidence-based approach, expertise in meniscal repair is a particularly important skill for every orthopaedic surgeon to possess. Successfully repairing a meniscus will have a major impact on the prognosis for subsequent development of arthritis, particularly in the younger, active patient. Surgeons should possess the knowledge to identify those meniscal tears which have the potential to heal, the skills necessary to achieve a stable repair, and the ability to advise patients on the appropriate rehabilitation to optimise the success of this surgery.

Focal loss of articular cartilage, either through injury or unexplained causes, remains a difficult challenge for the orthopaedic surgeon. Despite many years of research and clinical trials, and many worthwhile attempts at developing new products, there is still no reliable method to restore normal hyaline cartilage. Given that the first, seemingly promising, results of autologous chondrocyte implantation were reported nearly 30 years ago, it is somewhat disheartening that outcomes of current methods remain suboptimal and arguably not significantly superior to what was achieved 30 years ago. This therefore remains an area of ongoing study, and in planning any interventions intending to restore a cartilage surface, clinicians need to understand the pathology they are treating and its natural history, as well the risks, benefits, and likely outcomes of the treatment. Distinguishing between true focal lesions and early osteoarthritis is clearly critical when predicting natural history and the likely response to treatment. Introduction of any new technology needs to be done in a responsible, careful manner, with appropriate clinical trials prior to release to the general orthopaedic community. Chapter 5 has systematically reviewed the available options for management of this

problem, and this is clearly an area of orthopaedics that will continue to evolve, hopefully ultimately leading to a practical, easy-to-deliver solution for restoring a normal articular cartilage surface to these patients.

Osteotomy around the knee for osteoarthritis is a well-established procedure, predating joint replacement. Since the advent and increased popularity of joint replacement, osteotomy has been less commonly performed but remains a valuable option to consider for younger patients with well-localised, unicompartmental osteoarthritis. It offers the benefits of decreased pain and improved function, whilst not committing to the potential downside of arthroplasty in these patients. Osteotomy has also been shown to result in some cartilage recovery in diseased compartments, thereby having a positive effect on the natural history of osteoarthritis. The best results in osteotomy for osteoarthritis are in patients who have well-localised disease, correspondingly localised symptoms, and a joint that is not compromised by significant stiffness. Intervention prior to the more advanced stages of the disease is therefore preferable and will most likely yield better outcomes, but this needs to be balanced against the inconvenience of the procedure for the patient, particularly when they are not markedly symptomatic. Osteotomy is also an important supplement to procedures that may be used to restore chondral surfaces, in cases where this is associated with malalignment. When used for the appropriate indications, osteotomy is a procedure that can achieve excellent outcomes in the management of osteoarthritis, particularly in the younger patient group, and should be a procedure that all clinicians managing these patients are familiar with. Chapter 6 of this text has comprehensively addressed the various options for clinicians in the area of osteotomy.

Joint replacement comes in many forms, from focal resurfacing techniques to partial or total knee replacement. The common feature to all, however, is that the patient is committed to a prosthetic joint for the remainder of their life, with the accompanying potential limitations. Electing to perform a joint replacement is therefore a decision that should be made after considering and usually exhausting all other options, particularly in younger patients. What constitutes a "younger" patient is clearly somewhat arbitrary, but anyone under the age of 65 should be considered to have a reasonable chance of outliving their prosthesis and therefore not requiring revision surgery. In addition, there is a significant chance that younger patients, with higher expectations, may not find these expectations met by joint replacement in the same way that older patients with more modest expectations may. Whilst it should therefore always be considered a last resort for these patients, joint replacement does, however, offer a solution for those patients who have developed advanced arthritic change and for whom all alternative options have been trialled and subsequently found to be no longer effective. Performed in the right patient, with appropriate expectations, joint replacement can achieve excellent outcomes that should be sustained over long-term follow-up. Counselling patients about the limitations of joint replacement, and the appropriate level of activity they should expect postoperatively, is obviously critical in the management of these patients. Chapters 7 and 8 of this text have covered the role of joint replacement for these younger, active patients in detail and have provided clear guidelines about the appropriate application of these procedures.

So what does the future hold for the management of these patients? Clearly, there will always be new technologies being developed to try and address the growing problem, as enthusiasm from clinicians to better manage disease and the desire from industry to develop successful products continue to drive innovation. Chapter 9 of this text has covered some of the newer techniques being developed, but as with most new developments, they remain a work in progress and need to be carefully studied and evaluated as to their effectiveness before general application. Innovation needs to be supported and encouraged but with the appropriate balance of quality control and responsible introduction of new technology. Clearly, the ideal future lies in the prevention of osteoarthritis development in these patients, and there is certainly a great deal of investment currently aimed towards this goal, but it is safe to assume that this is a goal that is unlikely to be successfully achieved within most of our lifetimes.

Successful, effective management of osteoarthritis will therefore remain a major part of clinicians' practice in the years to come and requires an in-depth knowledge of both nonoperative and operative options for each patient, as outlined in this text. The necessary expertise to apply each treatment option in a coordinated, appropriately timed manner should be the domain of each clinician managing these patients. As the evidence base for these treatments grows, and clinicians base their management on this evidence, the overall management of these patients should improve. Ultimately, the goal should be to use this expertise to inform patients, as well as treat them effectively, with the result of a sustained improvement in the quality of life with minimal compromise from osteoarthritis.

Index

© ISAKOS 2016

D.A. Parker (ed.), *Management of Knee Osteoarthritis in the Younger, Active Patient:
An Evidence-Based Practical Guide for Clinicians*, DOI 10.1007/978-3-662-48530-9